This fascinating text achieves its intention of providing an accessible and informed perspective on the relationship between creativity and mental health recovery. The content is evocative and challenging and seeks to arouse the reader to explore their own relationship with creativity, whilst enabling the storyteller's narrative to explore how creativity has influenced their recovery. The authors' mutual respect for one another's lived experience is evident and provides a unique perspective.

**Annette Feakes** – *Senior Lecturer, University of Brighton*

This book shows how lived experiences constitute an invaluable source of knowledge. It is a book of showing and telling, and of making meaning of the past, present, and possible futures. These concepts are beautifully woven together through the tapestry that this book offers, demonstrating how creativity is something lived, personal and accessible, providing a powerful resource to mental health and well-being.

**Trude Klevan** – *Professor of Mental Health and Substance Use, University of South-Eastern Norway*

This book opens up exciting new vistas in understanding mental health recovery, by extending the Connectedness, Hope, Identity, Meaning and Empowerment (CHIME) Framework to incorporate the transformative and healing potential of Creativity (C-CHIME). Skillfully weaving individual accounts of how creative activities have impacted on recovery, a particular strength is the balanced focus both on benefits and possible harms. This book shows how creativity can bring light to the darkest of mental health experiences.

**Mike Slade** – *Professor of Mental Health Recovery and Social Inclusion, University of Nottingham*

I0025382

# Creative Mental Health Recovery

This book presents the importance of the role of creativity, particularly everyday creativity, in the lives of people on a mental health recovery journey.

Through a review of historical and contemporary literature and research findings on the topic, the book starts by giving readers an idea of the state of play of conceptualisations of both creativity and recovery. The authors arrive at and present their own definitions of these concepts, using autoethnography to bring their own experiences into the text. They then illustrate to the reader what creativity in recovery looks like in practice, through interviews with and written accounts from creative individuals who have experienced a mental health recovery journey, grounding the theory with tangible stories of application. The interviews are analysed, with themes picked out and a model of creativity and recovery produced by the authors. Implications and possible future directions are then discussed.

This unique presentation of creative recovery will be of interest to a wide range of mental health professionals, specifically those studying or practising mental health recovery and creative therapies.

**Robert Hurst** is an associate lecturer in the School of Psychology, University of Bolton. Alongside this, he is a practising person-centred counsellor, registered with the British Association for Counselling and Psychotherapy.

**Andrew Voyce** is a researcher and lived experience consultant. He is the author of several peer reviewed papers and two books. He has guest lectured on mental health recovery to a wide array of university students in the UK. In 2024, Andrew was awarded an honorary doctorate from the University of Bolton.

**Jerome Carson** is professor of psychology at the University of Bolton. A qualified clinical psychologist, Jerome's main research interests are mental health recovery, positive psychology, autoethnography, and alcohol addiction.

# Creative Mental Health Recovery

## An Approach to Healing

**Robert Hurst, Andrew Voyce, and Jerome Carson**

Routledge
Taylor & Francis Group

LONDON AND NEW YORK

Designed cover image: getty images © baani hakkam

First published 2025
by Routledge
4 Park Square, Milton Park, Abingdon, Oxon OX14 4RN

and by Routledge
605 Third Avenue, New York, NY 10158

*Routledge is an imprint of the Taylor & Francis Group, an informa business*

*British Library Cataloguing-in-Publication Data*
A catalogue record for this book is available from the British Library

ISBN: 9781032333717 (hbk)
ISBN: 9781032333687 (pbk)
ISBN: 9781003319405 (ebk)

DOI: 10.4324/9781003319405

Typeset in Times New Roman
by Newgen Publishing UK

Robert Hurst dedicates this book to the loving memory of Michael Russ, Patricia Russ and Jack Hurst. Wonderful Grandparents who fostered creativity and caring, all sorely missed each day. Andrew Voyce dedicates this book to Mum and Leonie. Jerome Carson dedicates this book to Cheryl.

# Contents

# Acknowledgements

I would firstly like to give thanks to my beautiful family, for all that they do. Particularly to my Mum, who is my hero and inspires me to always be kind and caring. To my Nana, for always having a place for me in her home and giving so much love. And of course to my brother, for joining in on all my daft adventures. They all offer a constant supply of love and support, and have always nurtured my creativity. For this, there are not words enough to thank them!

I am also blessed with a number of amazing friends and loved ones, who willingly listen to me talk at 100 miles per hour about my various ideas, and yet encourage my creative endeavours anyway. Special thanks to Heather, Izzy and Jack for all of their endless laughter, kindness, distraction and support. You always pick me up with so much love. Mention must also go to Danny, Josh, Courtney, Mithun, Ben, Jade, Nicola, Dana, Tony, Paul, Rachel, and Jess.

My workplace is full of excellent people. I thank Charlotte Conn, Aashiya Patel, Ana Tuluceanu, Linzi Robertson, and Dr Jack Brimmell for being constant founts of wisdom and for making me feel at home. I have appreciated the support and guidance of Prof Alec Grant as I navigate the world of autoethnography. Thanks also go to my uni buddy, Shahaa, for always pushing me to be my best academic self.

My work as a counsellor is foundational to my outlook on life, and subsequently my research and writing. In this regard, huge thanks go to Carole Darbyshire and Kevin Illingworth for supporting me not only as a counsellor, but as a person. They have helped shape my ideas, and I am a better person for knowing them. Also to my "Thursday Gang" – Neil, Dave, Christina, Sarah, and Nicole – for being such amazing people.

Huge thanks to Paul Meagher, for helping me to rediscover my creative spark.

Finally, to every friend, student, client, teacher, and colleague I have encountered for helping me to develop all of these ideas with all kinds of input, and for generally increasing, shifting, and challenging my worldview. I am lucky indeed.

Robert Hurst

I would like to acknowledge Margaret Moss who did so much to encourage me in writing my personal narrative, and Professor Jerome Carson for his substantial contribution to my recovery journey.

Andrew Voyce

The authors acknowledge the support of Professor Patrick McGhee, who provided a small amount of funding to enable us to carry out the five interviews and conduct this research on creativity.

Also we thank our editor Grace, for her support and understanding throughout the production of this work.

Jerome Carson

She asks *why don't you write*
*about me*? It's not that easy,
I tell her. Poetry is my therapist, sits
across the room with one finger
on its metaphorical lens,
says show me where you bleed.
 – Romina Ramos (@rominawrites),
   from the poem "*Metaphors For Falling In Love*".

# 1 Introduction

*Robert Hurst, Heather Harrison,*
*Andrew Voyce, and Jerome Carson*

Poland, 1944. As he enters Auschwitz concentration camp, Dr Viktor Frankl is forced to hand over a manuscript. It is his life's work. As he suffers unimaginable horrors (Frankl, 1985), one of the driving forces that pushes him to keep going is the hope that he will one day be able to publish his book. He goes over his ideas in his mind, constantly mentally rewriting sections of his manuscript so that he will not forget them. Scribbling frantic fragments on scraps of paper, stashing them out of sight from the guards.

Frankl was a psychiatrist, interested in meaning in life. His manuscript contained his ideas on the ways that meaning drives us forward in life. His experiences in the concentration camps of Europe strengthened and illustrated these ideas for him. However, his story can also be viewed as one of creativity.

During cold winter months, Dr Frankl passed the painful hours spent shovelling cold, hard earth by keeping his creative spark alight. Working on the confiscated manuscript in his mind was his own form of personal rebellion. He found ways to relate his academic ideas to his current experiences. He imagined a legacy for himself. It is an extreme example of what will be explored in this book – in what ways does creativity help us through our darkest days?

The links between creativity and wellbeing are well established. They pre-date psychology as an academic discipline.

## A brief history of creativity and wellbeing

### 1942

On February 15, 1942, the Allied army in Singapore surrendered to Japanese forces. 4,000 civilians were interned in Changi prison. Of them, 1,000 were women and children, separated from their adult male relatives for the remainder of the war. The dwellings were cramped and unhygienic, and the food was meagre (Archer, 1997). Anxieties emerged about whether loved ones had survived, about the threat of starvation and about the loss of identity. The response to these anxieties were acts of creation: the famous Changi quilt, and the lesser-known *Prisoner of War Cookbook*.

DOI: 10.4324/9781003319405-1

Both were overseen by Canadian prisoner Ethel Mulvaney, the unofficial Red Cross leader of the camp. She suggested that the women each create a six-inch square bearing her name and "something of herself". These squares would then be brought together into a quilt and sent across to a "craft fair" organised by the civilian men. The iconography is mainly a combination of "pretty" feminine motifs and national symbols: thistles and heather for Scotland, daffodils for Wales, shamrocks and harps for Ireland, maple leaves for Canada, and Union Jacks for Britain. Others made harrowing reference to their current captivity. Some mingled their loving icons with barbed wire imagery, or their cell number.

The women prisoners would also gather to recite recipes of their favourite meals and host imaginary dinners. These discussions inspired Mulvaney to write down the recipes, both simple and fantastical. Most of them are luxurious and complicated, with varying levels of skill required. It is not a recipe book designed to be followed. After the war ended, Ethel Mulvaney released her book, *Prisoner of War Cookbook: A Collection of Recipes Made by Starving Prisoners* (the exact publisher and year lost to time). She argued that not only did the sharing of recipes strengthen social relationships, but they also fostered a sense of hope that one day some of the women would be free to make the recipes they had learned. Mulvaney is quoted as writing "many of us slept with the feeling of having had a meal, after two or three hours of recipe writing" (Evans, 2013, p. 40).

It created a sense of identity in cramped conditions where diaries were banned. Canadian folklorist Diane Tye compared these pieces of writing to brief journal entries (Tye, 2010). They were acts of rebellion. A comparable claim is made about the recipes gathered by Mina Pachter, while she was imprisoned in Ravensbrück concentration camp. Culinary historian Cara De Silva thinks of these recipes as a collective memoir, which is "in some ways as revealing as prose" (De Silva, 1996, p. xl). The whimsical nature of the imaginary tea parties which inspired these cookbooks support writings on play within concentration camps. For prisoners "trapped in a chronic powerlessness, adult play represented an important escape and coping mechanism both in the emotional and mental realms" (Eisen, 1988, p. 72). Whereas children's play was about adjusting to reality, their elders found that "every means, among them play, had to be harnessed to provide badly needed counterbalances to the crippling effects of reality" (Eisen, 1988, p. 73). Creativity and play could provide a brief escape from the pain of imprisonment.

### *1569–1585*

Incarcerated in a very different way from the prisoners of 1940s Europe, in the latter half of the sixteenth century Mary Queen of Scots was imprisoned and isolated. Though she enjoyed a degree of luxury in well-furnished chambers maintained by her household staff, she was not allowed outside of these rooms without supervision. In this period, Mary, her domestic staff, and the wife of her jailer (Bess Hardwick), created over a hundred panels of embroidery together. Many of the panels feature Mary and Bess's monograms, as well as imagery of the natural world. The embroideries suggest that needlework was a powerful means of resistance during a period of constant surveillance. For example, one slip features a phoenix – a mythological creature capable of regeneration. In another, a crowned ginger cat toys with a grey mouse – a veiled representation of the unequal and uneasy relationship between herself and the red-haired Elizabeth Tudor. One panel displays a marigold (a name derived from "Mary's gold") turning towards the sun, suggesting hope in adversity. A yellow rose attacked by a group of caterpillars, suggesting a devouring feeling of despair (V&A, 2007). These panels are therefore a good example of hope, despair and identity being made into tangible items, by a small community working together.

### 1800s

Creativity is not only used to look towards the future, but is a method of processing the past. The creation of mourning objects gained great importance in American grieving processes in the nineteenth century. Examples of this include hair weavings, mourning quilts, mourning portraits, and consolation poems (Bradford, 2014). Their purpose was to maintain "affective attachments" with the dead; they are a physical manifestation of continuing bonds with the deceased (Klass et al., 2014).

Arlonzia Pettway described how she assisted her mother in creating a mourning quilt for her father:

> It was when Daddy died. I was about seventeen, eighteen. He stayed sick about eight months and passed on. Mama say, "I going to take his work clothes, shape them into a quilt to remember him, and cover up under it for love." She take his old pants legs and shirttails, take all the clothes he had, just enough to make that quilt, and I helped her tore them up. Bottom of the pants is narrow, top is wide, and she had me to cutting the top part out and to shape them up in even strips.
>
> (Collins, 2015, p. 345)

Again, it is an example of collaborative creation, which in this example served to counter Arlonzia's drive to alienate herself in her grief.

### 1987

Such practices were not restricted to the nineteenth century. In San Francisco, 1987, the NAMES Project began as a way of memorialising those who had died of acquired immunodeficiency syndrome (AIDS). Since the first cases were reported 40 years ago, more than 700,000 lives have been lost to the disease. The project's AIDS Memorial Quilt has nearly 110,000 names sewn into its panels, and weighs 54 tons (National AIDS Memorial, n.d.). Its aim was to counter the anonymity of those who had died privately, to show the scale of the losses while maintaining the memory of individuals. As of 2020, it is the largest example of community folk art in the world. A massive outpouring of grief. A huge attempt to heal through creation.

Evidently the idea that creativity can have a positive impact on mental health is nothing new. Nor is it novel. So, what is this book hoping to add?

## Aims of the book

Broadly, this book aims to inspire conversation about the role that creativity plays in mental health recovery. We the authors find the concepts of both creativity and recovery to be fuzzy in their current definitions. We aim to present a range of these to the reader, before introducing our own attempt at conceptualising them. Our method for doing this was through qualitative research – talking to people.

We are conscious that ideas cannot and should not come only from the minds of academics. We have spoken to five people about their experiences of creativity in mental health recovery. Their stories are key to this book, an emotional foundation. Splashes of reality. We will explain the research that we undertook with these five people, share their stories, and produce a novel conception of creativity in recovery from them.

Above all else, we aim to make this book as accessible as we can. It is an academic text, and you will find citations throughout it. However, we want to write in a way that intrigues and engages with as many people as possible. We hope that anybody who picks up this book will be able to understand us.

## Who are you?

As you continue to turn the pages, you will get to know your three lead authors in greater detail. However, now seems a good time to briefly introduce ourselves.

Professor Jerome Carson sparked the idea for this project. His wisdom from 27 years as a clinical psychologist in the NHS has been invaluable. He has seen people in distress. He has seen several of them recover. Currently, he is Professor of Psychology at the University of Bolton. Co-writing first-hand recovery narratives with students (e.g. Jenkins & Carson, 2014), he has unearthed a lot about what is involved in recovery.

Andrew Voyce is the most experienced of the three of us. He had a 17-year career as a "revolving door mental patient". After a diagnosis of schizophrenia in 1975, Andrew spent years between various hospitals. This included time in the asylums before they were shut down around the early 1990s. After a number of years living in bus shelters, Andrew found his own path to recovery. His story is remarkable, and you will hear more of it later. In this project, he has provided a grounding in lived experience, ensuring that we are on the right tracks. That we are considering things that we might not otherwise think of.

Robert Hurst is the creative force. It is in his voice that you will read the majority of this book. This project is dear to him, this book being the culmination of months of hard work, and years of being drawn to the power of creativity. He brings a drive and passion to this book. As well as being a researcher, Robert is a counsellor. He cares about helping people to heal. If this book can give practitioners and those with lived experience some ideas about how that might happen, he will be happy. Above all, he wants it to be kind and considered.

## Key terms

Throughout the book, we will be using language carefully. Words are powerful (Granello & Gibbs, 2016). They can help, and they can harm. Throughout the text of this book, each word is chosen and used with the best of intentions. If we use a word that does not make sense to you and your own experiences, we are sorry. It can be hard to find a term that works for everybody.

Recovery is a slippery term (Ellison et al., 2018). It means a great many things to various people. Indeed, it is used in many contexts, including addiction (Ogilvie & Carson, 2022). For clarity, in this text "recovery" always refers to "mental health recovery".

The concept of recovery and its origins will be further explored in Chapter 2. However, a brief summary would be that when somebody experiences psychological distress, or what is often referred to as "a mental illness", recovery is a journey back to "wellbeing". For many readers we are sure that the inherent issues with this term are obvious. How do we define "illness"? How do we define "wellness"? Is "recovery" really the best word to describe the journey from one state to the other (Piat et al., 2008)? The people we spoke to for this book seem to think not. All five of them were uncomfortable using the word "recovery" to describe their own experiences. It didn't fit their story. Some preferred "discovery", seeing the journey as a navigation of new information. You discover lots about yourself and the world, and learn in time how to balance the two.

So, is "recovery" the right word? Perhaps not. It can be perceived that recovery is a word "coming from higher above" (Aston & Coffey, 2012, p. 260), as it is created and maintained by various stakeholders – whether they be academics or policy makers (e.g. Jacobson, 2003). Though service users may be consulted (Wallcraft et al., 2011), we must acknowledge that it is, ultimately, a top-down construct with financial stakes involved. However, the majority of academic therapeutic literature *does* define this huge, foundational concept as "recovery". And, when studied and applied with care, it is an important concept! It needs to be called something. Some kind of banner under which to gather. It will have to do for now.

On the topic of psychological distress, now is a good time to explain to readers that they will not see the words "mental illness" used in the book. While the term seems to be commonly accepted, widespread even, we feel that it represents a dated idea. Part of the recovery movement is to move away from a medicalised view of recovery. "Mental illness" is a hangover from this medical approach to treating psychological pain as if it were physical.

As Peter Bullimore puts it in Chapter 8: "I wasn't ill. What happened to me was a consequence of my life experiences." The factors that might lead to receiving a label from a doctor (depression, anxiety, etc.) are incredibly complex in their causes. There may be a genetic or biological element (Alameda et al., 2022).

Perhaps the symptoms are trauma-related (Rafiq et al., 2018), or they may even be due to a disruption of circadian rhythms (Jones & Benca, 2015). We lump these experiences under labels because it helps us to treat negative symptoms (Grant, 2015). Because they help us to share briefly with others the general gist of our distress. However, they do not, to our minds, represent a set category. An "illness" that can be "treated".

In disability literature, Simplican (2015) wrote that a medical model is appealing because it eases the anxiety of "able-bodied" individuals. We may look at this through the lens of mental health, substituting "able-bodied" for "mentally well". Medicalisation creates a category – "mentally ill" – which is separate. In this way, the term makes individuals become "other". "Well" individuals have no reason to worry about social injustices, as those others are just "ill". It also eases the anxieties of "well" people, as they have less cause for concern at becoming "ill", as "illness" is something other and apart from them. This binary is, of course, ridiculous. Short and Grant (2016) critiqued the reliance of recovery services on distancing professionals from service user via this rigid "ill/well" binary.

So, we echo the words of esteemed mental health advocacy writer Patricia Deegan – "We are refusing to reduce human beings to illnesses" (Deegan, 1996b).

Instead, the terminology we will use to describe this phenomenon, inspired by Llewellyn-Beardsley et al. (2022), is "people with lived experience of mental distress". For brevity, this will usually be phrased as simply "lived experience" or "mental health difficulties". We hope that this is more humanising and encapsulates the experiences of the most people possible.

Now onto the people who have shaped this book. The five individuals whom you will come to know in Chapters 6–10 took part in a research project with us that formed the basis of this book (more on that in Chapter 5). Commonly in research, helpful individuals like our five are referred to as "participants". This word serves a purpose. They did indeed participate in research. Yet, this feels rather clinical. This is not a clinical book. It is about creativity. We see these five people as much more than just numbers and anonymous acronyms in a study. We may have written the research, but they *made* it. By sharing their experiences, they shaped the directions that the research took and informed our conceptualisations of creativity in recovery. As such, we are giving them the moniker "StoryTellers". We humans are shaped by stories, they are how we communicate (Storr, 2019). We considered "Narrators", to match the common term "recovery narratives" (Woods et al., 2022). However, we feel that "StoryTellers" lends an air of wisdom which our five certainly possess.

**Key concepts**

One of the other key concepts running through the book is that of "autoethnography". This is, in essence, an academic way of saying that we will be bringing some of our own experiences in at points in the book where it is pertinent to illustrate an academic point with a real, emotive, lived-in example. This will hopefully help readers better understand what we are talking about, and perhaps give them a chance to reflect on their own experiences. The word autoethnography is an amalgamation of "auto-" and "ethnography", the latter being a well-established methodology in various fields. In ethnography, a researcher places themselves in a social group in order to better understand functions within that group. So *auto*ethnography is where, through reflection, you try to make sense of your self, and the place that you inhabit in the social world. Ethnography itself breaks down to two words, which gives us a full breakdown of "auto-", "ethno-" and "-graphy". To translate into plain English, these mean the self, the social, and the study of these (Adams & Herrmann, 2020). Those are the three defining factors of autoethnography.

Some might call this mode of writing "creative non-fiction". They wouldn't necessarily be wrong. All three of us have experience writing autoethnography (Carson & Niklasson, 2023; Hurst & Carson, 2021; Voyce & Carson, 2020). The way it appears in this book will be rather different from that, though. Perhaps it is one massive, collaborative autoethnography. It concerns the stories of three Researchers, and also the stories of our five StoryTellers. That means that the product of this work is down to at least 8 people. Their stories interweave and bounce off each other to create one narrative and ultimately a new conceptualisation of creativity in recovery. It is important for us to bring our stories into this. To share what motivated us to carry out all of the work that went into this book. We shaped the project just like the StoryTellers did. While some books would hide that, we want to share it with the reader. To allow you to notice what might be blind spots for us. For you to get a sense of why we understood the literature and the narratives of the StoryTellers in the way that we did. It provides greater perspective. Is it naval gazing (Ellis, 2009)? We think not. Sharing narratives around recovery can reduce feelings of stigma and increase readers' understandings (Rennick-Egglestone et al., 2019), which meets our aims for this project. However, don't take our word for it. We encourage you to draw your own conclusions!

That is the final key concept. This text is not a definitive guide to recovery. Nor is it a comprehensive text on creativity. It is a presentation of where we believe these two concepts currently are, and how they might be missing the mark. It is an exploration of the misunderstandings around how creativity can help to heal. It is illustrated through story, through emotions and experiences. There are no huge datasets to back it up. We are not convinced that there should be. We aim to write in an evocative way (Bochner & Ellis, 2016). We want to make you think. To present you with stories from the past, a picture of the present, and propose a better way forward.

This project was a journey. Think of this book as more of a travel book. Join us. We will make many stops along the way. Describe places so you need not go there yourself. But create intrigue, give you a sense of where you would like to go. Of what is pleasant, and what is scary. Read the book, but do not think it is gospel. You have been on your own travels, no doubt. Author your own story. As you read, fit it into ours. Decide what works and what doesn't, whether that is for your practice or for your own recovery journey. Then talk about it. In a safe way, of course, but discuss it with others. What we desire from our writing is conversation. Think critically about how creativity is portrayed. Live with your own definition.

**What is in the book?**

To help you get a feel of what is to come, we will now briefly outline the chapters in this book. In this first chapter, you have seen us introduce the concept of creativity and how it has always been used by individuals to adapt to adversity. We have explained some of the concepts behind this book, and what we aim to achieve with it. The three co-editors of the book have been introduced, and some of the terminology that we will be using has been explained. This chapter features an extra co-author – our historical helper, Heather Harrison, who helped weave a tapestry for the readers of the ways in which creativity has been used by individuals to influence their mental health for millennia.

Chapter 2 focuses on the origins of recovery as a concept. Jerome first encountered recovery when he heard American clinical psychologist Patricia Deegan at a World Psychiatric Rehabilitation Congress in Rotterdam (Deegan, 1996a). It was to be a further decade before Jerome began to become genuinely involved with the recovery movement. In this chapter he tells of his journey, the people he met along the way, and current thinking on recovery.

Chapter 3 is a deep dive into a framework of recovery that has influenced this project greatly. The Connectedness, Hope and optimism, Identity, Meaning and Empowerment (CHIME) framework is examined, including the ways in which it has been applied by helping professionals. Then, some work by Robert and Jerome is shared which utilised CHIME, before arguing for it to be expanded to include creativity.

Chapter 4 picks up this thread and looks more closely at creativity and its blurry definitions. Issues around gatekeeping and potentially damaging conceptualisations are examined. Robert explores how creativity has been applied clinically to help people, and how perhaps it is something that each of us actually does every single day.

Chapter 5 is the most obviously autoethnographic chapter. The three of us discuss what drew us to this project, our encounters with creativity and recovery. We ask you to reflect on the way you use creativity in your life. Finally, we outline the research project that spawned this book. We tell you how we gathered our stories and explain how we will then present them.

Chapters 6–10 are our StoryTeller chapters. In each, Robert sets the scene, before allowing the gems of this project to shine – the stories of five real individuals. In Chapter 6, Jo Mullen gives us a solid theoretical and philosophical grounding in both creativity and recovery as she sees them. Michelle McNary in Chapter 7 shows us that creativity is not always positive – it can be a double-edged sword. Chapter 8 sees Peter Bullimore beautifully illustrate creativity in action. In Chapter 9, ANON gives us insight into how being creative for work can impact mental health. Finally, Anna Sexton shares with us tales of stitching and re-storying in Chapter 10.

Chapter 11 is Andrew Voyce's own StoryTeller chapter. He talks about the massive healing impact that creativity has had on him, as well as the power of collaboration. His writing is personal, but also draws on literature.

In Chapter 12, Robert attempts to pull everything that has gone before into a cohesive idea of creativity in mental health recovery. Drawing upon concepts of recovery, rallying against some ideas of creativity, and utilising the words of the StoryTellers, Robert creates a model and illustrates how creativity can be added to CHIME to make C-CHIME.

Finally, Chapter 13 sees us ask where this leaves us. What can we learn from the StoryTellers and the C-CHIME framework? What positive changes could be made to better help those recovering to harness the healing power of creativity?

## References

Adams, T. E., & Herrmann, A. F. (2020). Expanding our autoethnographic future. *Journal of Autoethnography, 1*(*1*), 1–8. doi:10.1525/joae.2020.1.1.1.

Alameda, L., Trotta, G., Quigley, H., Rodriguez, V., Gadelrab, R., Dwir, D., … & Di Forti, M. (2022). Can epigenetics shine a light on the biological pathways underlying major mental disorders? *Psychological Medicine, 52*(*9*), 1645–1665. doi:10.1017/S0033291721005559.

Archer, B. (1997). A patchwork of internment. *History Today, 47*(*7*), 11–19. https://go.gale.com/ps/i.do?id=GALE%7CA19581006&sid=googleScholar&v=2.1&it=r&linkaccess=abs&issn=00182753&p=AONE&sw=w&userGroupName=anon%7E6eee0644.

Aston, V., & Coffey, M. (2012). Recovery: What mental health nurses and service users say about the concept of recovery. *Journal of Psychiatric and Mental Health Nursing, 19*(*3*), 257–263. doi:10.1111/j.1365-2850.2011.01776.x.

Bochner, A. & Ellis, C. (2016). *Evocative autoethnography: Writing lives and telling stories.* Routledge.

Bradford, A. C. (2014). *Communities of death: Whitman, Poe, and the American culture of mourning.* University of Missouri Press.

Carson, J. & Niklasson, M. (2023). The struggle to get a PhD: The collaborative autoethnographic accounts of two "journeymen". *Journal of Further and Higher Education, 47*(*5*), 607–618. doi:10.1080/0309877X.2023.2222363.

Collins, L. G. (2015). Cycles of mourning and memory: Quilts by mother and daughter in Gee's Bend, Alabama. *The Journal of the History of Childhood and Youth 8*(*3*), 345–352. doi:10.1353/hcy.2015.0039.

De Silva, C. (1996). *In memory's kitchen: A legacy from the women of Terezin* (B. S. Brown, trans.). Jason Aronson.

Deegan, P. (1996a). Recovery as a journey of the heart. *Psychiatric Rehabilitation Journal, 19*(*3*), 91. doi:10.1037/h0101301.

Deegan, P. (1996b). *Recovery and the conspiracy of hope.* Speech presented at "There's a Person in Here": The Sixth Annual Mental Health Services Conference of Australia and New Zealand, Brisbane, Australia.

Eisen, G. (1988). *On children and play in the Holocaust: Games among the shadows.* University of Massachusetts Press.

Ellis, C. (2009). Fighting back or moving on: An autoethnographic response to critics. *International Review of Qualitative Research, 2*(*3*), 371–378. doi:10.1525/irqr.2009.2.3.371.

Ellison, M. L., Belanger, L. K., Niles, B. L., Evans, L. C., & Bauer, M. S. (2018). Explication and definition of mental health recovery: A systematic review. *Administration and Policy* in *Mental Health and Mental Health Services Research*, *45*(*1*), 91–102. doi:10.1007/s10488-016-0767-9.

Evans, S. (2013). Culinary imagination as a survival tool: Ethel Mulvany and the Changi Jail Prisoners of War Cookbook, Singapore, 1942–1945. *Canadian Military History*, *22*(*1*), 39–49. https://scholars.wlu.ca/cgi/viewcontent.cgi?article=1680&context=cmh.

Frankl, V. E. (1985). *Man's search for meaning*. Simon & Schuster.

Granello, D. H., & Gibbs, T. A. (2016). The power of language and labels: "The mentally ill" versus "people with mental illnesses". *Journal of Counseling & Development*, *94*(*1*), 31–40. doi:10.1002/jcad.12059.

Grant, A. (2015). Demedicalising misery: Welcoming the human paradigm in mental health nurse education. *Nurse Education Today*, *35*(*9*), e50–e53. doi:10.1016/j.nedt.2015.05.022.

Hurst, R., & Carson, J. (2021). Be honest, why did YOU decide to study psychology? A recent graduate and a professor reflect. *Psychology Teaching Review*, *27*(*2*), 22–35.

Jacobson, N. (2003). Defining recovery: An interactionist analysis of mental health policy development, Wisconsin 1996–1999. *Qualitative Health Research*, *13*(*3*), 378–393. doi:10.1177/1049732302250334.

Jenkins, C., & Carson, J. (2014). Remarkable lives: Caitlin Jenkins in conversation with Jerome Carson. *Mental Health and Social Inclusion*, *18*(*4*), 180–184. doi:10.1108/MHSI-08-2014-0031.

Jones, S. G., & Benca, R. M. (2015). Circadian disruption in psychiatric disorders. *Sleep Medicine Clinics*, *10*(*4*), 481–493. doi:10.1016/j.jsmc.2015.07.004.

Klass, D., Silverman, P. R., & Nickman, S. (2014). *Continuing bonds: New understandings of grief*. Taylor & Francis.

Llewellyn-Beardsley, J., Rennick-Egglestone, S., Pollock, K., Ali, Y., Watson, E., Franklin, D., Yeo, C., Ng, F., McGranahan, R., Slade, M., & Edgley, A. (2022). 'Maybe I shouldn't talk': The role of power in the telling of mental health recovery stories. *Qualitative Health Research*, *32*(*12*), 1828–1842. doi:10.1177/10497323221118239.

National AIDS Memorial. (n.d.). The history of the quilt. Retrieved 10 December 2022 from www.aidsmemorial.org/quilt-history.

Ogilvie, L., & Carson, J. (2022). Trauma, stages of change and post traumatic growth in addiction: A new synthesis. *Journal of Substance Use*, *27*(*2*), 122–127. doi:10.1080/14659891.2021.1905093.

Piat, M., Sabetti, J., & Couture, A. (2008). Do consumers use the word "Recovery"? *Psychiatric Services*, *59*(*4*), 446–447. doi:10.1176/ps.2008.59.4.446.

Rafiq, S., Campodonico, C., & Varese, F. (2018). The relationship between childhood adversities and dissociation in severe mental illness: A meta-analytic review. *Acta Psychiatrica Scandinavica*, *138*(*6*), 509–525. doi:10.1111/acps.12969.

Rennick-Egglestone, S., Morgan, K., Llewellyn-Beardsley, J., Ramsay, A., McGranahan, R., Gillard, S., … & Slade, M. (2019). Mental health recovery narratives and their impact on recipients: Systematic review and narrative synthesis. *The Canadian Journal of Psychiatry*, *64*(*10*), 669–679. doi:10.1177/0706743719846108.

Short, N. P., & Grant, A. (2016). Poetry as hybrid pedagogy in mental health nurse education. *Nurse Education Today*, *43*, 60–63. doi:10.1016/j.nedt.2016.05.003.

Simplican, S. C. (2015). *The capacity contract: Intellectual disability and the question of citizenship*. University of Minnesota Press.

Storr, W. (2019). *The science of storytelling*. William Collins.

Tye, D. (2010). *Baking as biography: A life story in recipes*. McGill-Queen's University Press.

V&A. (2007). The Marian hanging. https://collections.vam.ac.uk/item/O137608/the-marian-hanging-hanging-mary-queen-of/.

Voyce, A., & Carson, J. (2020). Our lives in three parts: An autoethnographic account of two undergraduates and their respective psychiatric careers. *Mental Health and Social Inclusion, 24*(*4*), 197–205. doi:10.1108/MHSI-07-2020-0045.

Wallcraft, J. A. N., Amering, M., Freidin, J., Davar, B., Froggatt, D., Jafri, H., ... & Herrman, H. (2011). Partnerships for better mental health worldwide: WPA recommendations on best practices in working with service users and family carers. *World Psychiatry, 10*(*3*), 229–236. doi:10.1002/j.2051-5545.2011.tb00062.x.

Woods, A., Hart, A., & Spandler, H. (2022). The recovery narrative: Politics and possibilities of a genre. *Culture, Medicine, and Psychiatry, 46*(*2*), 221–247. doi:10.1007/s11013-019-09623-y.

# 2    Recovery journeys in mental health

*Jerome Carson*

When the pupil is ready the teacher will appear.

(Buddhist saying)

### From the clinic to the classroom

I am now a teacher. I arrived in the town of Bolton in September 2012 to become professor of psychology at the University of Bolton. I assumed that I would be able to educate the students about mental health problems, having spent 32 years in the National Health Service working in psychiatry. I wanted to bring the clinic into the classroom, as I had done previously in an adult education setting (Carson & Brewerton, 1991). I soon discovered the clinic was already in the classroom. That is, many of the students I was teaching had mental health problems themselves. In a paper I co-authored with Robert (Hurst & Carson, 2021), I suggested that I probably chose to study psychology for unconscious reasons. I became a wounded healer who never even realised he was wounded (Rippere & Williams, 1985).

At the time of writing I am 66 years old. I have entered a much more reflective period of my life. As an academic, I have to be able to articulate my specific research interests many times when applying for grants, etc. My main research interests are positive psychology, alcohol addiction, bereavement, positive aging, autoethnography, and, most importantly, mental health recovery. I read the acknowledgements section of a book once which stated, "If you don't see your name in this section, it is because your role was not as important as you thought it was!" A sobering thought. If you should look at the Scopus "Researcher Discovery" section using the term "mental health recovery", you will find that I am not in the Top 10 recovery researchers worldwide. If you instead put in the terms, "mental health illness recovery", you will see that in February 2024, I was the eighth most productive researcher in this field since 2020. "Lies, damned lies, and statistics!" Why does this matter? It matters because I believe all of us wants to feel that we have made an impact on the world. A participant in one of my "Enhancing self-esteem" workshops (Carson, 2006) commented, "We are born, we die, it's what we do in between that counts". Professor John Strauss, talking about a patient he had got to know during a longitudinal research project, quoted him saying, "I always

DOI: 10.4324/9781003319405-2

wanted to leave this world a little better than I found it". Robert raises the existential question of life's meaning in Chapter 1, drawing on the work of Viktor Frankl. I have recently "raised eyebrows" by quoting the words from the song by Billie Eilish from the movie Barbie – "What was I made for?". It is a question for all of us. What is the purpose of each of our lives? What were we made for?

## CHIME and its variations

In Chapter 1, Heather Harrison gave us a short history of creativity. She cited examples like the AIDS quilt and the prisoner cookbook. In Chapter 4, Robert explores definitions of creativity. In Chapter 3, he looks in depth at the CHIME framework of mental health recovery. This framework has become dominant in the research literature. To borrow a quotation from Lord of the Rings, "One ring to rule them all". Robert and I had earlier suggested that the framework be expanded to C-CHIME (Carson & Hurst, 2021). Lisa Ogilvie and I had offered G-CHIME as a framework for addiction recovery, "G" representing growth (Ogilvie & Carson, 2023). More recently one of my PhD students, Ije Asike, has been trying to develop PAA-CHIME for sufferers of lupus. The "P" representing pain, the "A" Acceptance and the second "A" Adaptation. I am currently working with Julie Fletcher and Dr Trish Houghton on how the CHIME framework might be applied to nurses, Professional CHIME or P-CHIME for short. But where did the actual concept of recovery come from. What was there before the development of the CHIME framework?

## The history of mental health recovery

As I note in Chapter 5, I was involved with Michelle McNary (see her story in Chapter 7), in making a film about mental health recovery (Carson et al., 2012; Maudsley NHS, 2010). To accompany the film, I co-edited a short series of papers entitled "Recovery journeys: Stories of coping with mental health problems" (Carson et al., 2008). This featured narratives from the four central characters in the film, Dolly Sen, Gordon McManus, James Bellamy, and Ben Haydon. It also had stories from the filmmaker Michelle McNary, and Dr Paul Wolfson, who helped with the script and in auditioning people for the film. The book also had an account from the rehabilitation psychiatrist, Dr Frank Holloway, on his perspective on the history of recovery.

Frank chose nine sets of authors to illustrate how the concept of recovery had evolved over two centuries. He started with the York Retreat and the work of William Tuke. He commented that this offered "humane treatment in homely circumstances, where people were offered hope ... building on their strengths" (Holloway, 2008, p. 5). He then talked about four major influences from the United States. The first of these was the work of the mental health activist Judi Chamberlin. The second was the psychiatrist and anthropologist Richard Warner. He observed that low rates of recovery from mental health problems were related to social and cultural factors and not to advances in psychopharmacology. The third was the work of Larry Davidson and John Strauss. They stressed the importance of the person's re-discovery of a sense of self as an active and responsible agent. His fourth source was the inspirational Pat Deegan, of whom more later.

He then turned to the British psychiatrist David Whitwell, who questioned whether anyone really recovers. His argument was that we never really go back to how we were earlier in life. We are constantly changing. He was also impressed with the work of the New Zealand based activist, Mary O'Hagan. She defined recovery as "the ability to live well in the presence or absence of one's mental illness (or whatever people choose to name that experience). Each person needs to define for themselves what living well means to them" (Holloway, 2008, p. 6).

He ends his short history of recovery with two further English sources. Repper and Perkins (2003) cite a triad of fostering hope, giving people a sense of control over their lives, and offering people opportunities to access roles, relationships and activities that are important to them. Rachel Perkins has summarised this elsewhere as people needing "Somewhere to live, something to do and someone to love". It sounds simple, but in practice many people with mental health problems will sadly be unemployed and not have a life partner. The final paper he cites is a policy paper from the Care Services Improvement Partnership (CSIP, 2007), which speculates about the future of recovery in mental health services. It predicted that it would be unlikely there would be a single model of recovery. The CHIME framework had not been developed at that point. So how should we then define mental health recovery?

### Defining recovery

The most widely cited definition of recovery is that of the late American psychologist Professor Bill Anthony. He described it thus:

> Recovery is … a deeply personal, unique process of changing one's attitudes, values, feelings, goals, skills, and/or roles. It is a way of living a satisfying, hopeful, and contributing life even with limitations caused by illness. Recovery involves the development of new meaning and purpose in one's life as one grows beyond the catastrophic effects of mental illness.
>
> (Anthony, 1993, p. 15)

There are of course many other definitions, but the most succinct to my mind is that provided by Gordon McManus. Gordon stated that "Recovery is coping with your illness, and having a meaningful life" (McManus et al., 2009). This combines the two types of recovery denoted by Professor Mike Slade, of clinical and personal recovery (Slade, 2009), and more recently repurposed as "professional-directed treatment" and "person-directed treatment" (Khan & Tracy, 2022). In an earlier paper, Carson et al. (2010), we attempted to identify the top 10 recovery papers, policy papers, books, and websites. Repeating a similar exercise today we might add the top 10 recovery films, such as the film *A Beautiful Mind*, about the life of the mathematician John Nash.

In teaching students about recovery, I try to get across this notion of professionals and people with lived experience working together. I have a slide that features three people. On one side there is a photo of me, taken at my NHS retirement in 2011 at Guy's Hospital. On the opposite side of the photo, there is a picture of Matt Ward at the same event. Matt was asked by his occupational therapist to approach me and ask what he could do for our Recovery Group. Matt was an actor who had been diagnosed with bipolar disorder. This meeting marked the start of what was to be an amazing relationship, which reached its zenith when Matt performed the one-man play *St Nicholas* in Governor's Hall, at St Thomas' Hospital. In between Matt and I was the clinical psychologist, Dr Rachel Perkins. Like Matt, Rachel also has lived experience of bipolar disorder (Perkins, 1999). She is what the Americans call a "prosumer". That is a professional who "consumes" mental health services. Our understanding of the difficulties faced by people with major mental health problems, has been greatly enriched by Rachel, especially her inspirational work around employment. The other "prosumer" who has had an equally dramatic effect on this field, is Dr Patricia Deegan, also a clinical psychologist. Pat had been admitted to psychiatric hospital three times by the time she was 18 yet went on later to become a clinical psychologist. To my mind she has written the greatest ever paper on recovery: "Recovery as a journey of the heart" (Deegan, 1996). I am now going to analyse her paper in search of the C-CHIME framework, to see if her own story maps onto this framework.

## Pat Deegan and the C-CHIME framework

### Creativity

Deegan's (1996) paper is of course an act of creativity on its own. It is based around a metaphor of the human heart. "Just as the generic, anatomical heart does not exist … what exists is a human being … Wisdom demands we … enter into a relationship with human beings in order to understand their experience" (Deegan, 1996, p. 92). Deegan exploits the use of this metaphor very effectively throughout the paper.

### Connectedness

"I had a strong therapeutic alliance with a psychotherapist" (Deegan, 1996, p. 96). What she commented on in the video but not in the paper, was that this person really believed in her. In the paper she notes, "the people around me did not give up on me. They kept inviting me to do things" (p. 96). The human interactive relationship may well be the most powerful factor in recovery.

### Hope

Deegan draws on Seligman's learned helplessness. She comments, "in an effort to avoid the biologically disastrous effects of profound helplessness, people with disabilities ... grow hard of heart and attempt to stop caring. It is safer to become helpless than to become hopeless" (Deegan, 1996, p. 94). This I feel is one of the most important insights from this paper. Seligman's model was initially put forward as a possible model for "reactive" depression, but Deegan uses it very effectively in developing our understanding of why people with mental health difficulties may appear "unmotivated". She was also determined to resist the negativity that had been expressed to her. A psychiatrist once said to her, "If you take medications for the rest of your life and avoid stress, then maybe you can cope" (p. 92). This, she said was a "prognosis of doom". She was able to use the "angry indignation" this stirred up in her as a positive, which gave her the motivation to move forward. In more contemporary terminology this could be seen as the positive power of negative emotions (Lomas, 2016). Hope for Deegan is central to recovery.

### Identity

"I decided that I wanted to get a powerful degree and have enough credentials to run a healing place myself" (Deegan, 1996, p. 96). "I was planning on getting my PhD in clinical psychology" (p. 96). She felt that this would give her the ability to change the mental health system. Almost 20 years on it would be interesting to find out if she felt she achieved this.

### Meaning

> I had a strong spirituality ... When I got out of bed in the morning, I always knew the reason why I had a purpose in life, I had been called, I had a vocation and I kept saying yes to it.
>
> (Deegan, 1996, p. 96)

It would be interesting to understand more about this. Was it her negative experiences of psychiatric services in her mid to late teenage years, which helped her identify that the area of mental health was one that she wanted to do something about, and have this as her life's mission?

### Empowerment

"I somehow intuited that drugs and alcohol were bad news for me ... I read tons of books about healing and psychopathology in an effort to understand myself and my situation" (Deegan, 1996, p. 96). In fact, she went on to establish the first National Empowerment Centre in Lawrence, Massachusetts.

Patricia Deegan's story is the most inspirational recovery account that I have ever come across, it also embodies the CHIME framework, which Robert will explore in more depth in the next chapter.

**Consolidated framework for recovery**

Gyanfi et al. (2022) have tried to distil wisdom from the CHIME framework, along with other recovery frameworks, into what they refer to as a "consolidated framework for recovery-oriented services", which they propose has three main elements. The first is "Mechanisms and strategies". These could include formal therapeutic interventions, such as cognitive behavioural therapy, exercise, medication, diet, and spirituality. The second is "Internal recovery", which covers processes like self-understanding, self-acceptance, self-control, and self-belief. "External recovery", the third element, covers social support, responsive mental health services, appropriate housing, occupation, arts programmes, and income. They argue that their approach is the first to provide a unified framework of recovery concepts. This is however a "top-down" approach and one that does not seem to have involved the participation of people who use mental health services or have lived experience.

**Conclusions**

It was in 1996 that I first came across Patricia Deegan at the World Psychiatric Rehabilitation Congress in Rotterdam. She was a keynote speaker in a symposium which included the American psychiatrist, Professor John Strauss. By the end I was so impressed by it that I bought her video! I must have watched that video over 100 times. I used it in training sessions and also in my work with individual clients, alongside her paper (Deegan, 1996). It was not until 2006 that I started to seriously incorporate the recovery approach into my clinical practice. Deegan's notion of seeing the patient as a hero was the inspiration for our series of Recovery Heroes, which led onto Remarkable Lives (Davies et al., 2011). The Remarkable Lives series in now curated by Robert. It also inspired our book, *Psychosis Stories of Recovery and Hope* (Cordle et al., 2011). I used the recovery approach with groups (Morgan & Carson, 2009), with individuals (McManus & Carson, 2012), and with communities (Ward et al., 2010).

Along the way, I have developed close friendships with Peter Bullimore and Andrew Voyce, two of Britain's leading lived experience experts. I may well have co-authored more books and papers with people who have lived experience of recovery than any other mental health professional. In 2006, when I was asked to leave the Institute of Psychiatry because of my lack of publications, I had reached a nadir. Yet, this signalled a re-birth and a re-discovery of recovery (Roberts & Wolfson, 2004). Little did I know then that this was to help my own recovery from the disappointment of losing my clinical academic position. I then embarked on a journey meeting some of the most amazing individuals who were all battling long-term mental health problems. Sir Isaac Newton once said, "If I have seen further, it is because I have stood on the shoulder of giants". I have been privileged to have met and worked with many "giants" of the recovery field. These have included Dolly Sen, Michelle McNary, Peter Chadwick, Matt Ward, Stuart Baker-Brown, James Bellamy, Liz Wakely, Gordon McManus, and numerous other amazing individuals. Too many to mention. Each of these people has not only enriched my own journey of professional recovery, but they have also touched my heart and soul.

## References

Anthony, W. A. (1993). Recovery from mental illness: The guiding vision of the mental health service system in the 1990s. *Psychosocial Rehabilitation Journal, 16*(*4*), 11–23. doi:10.1037/h0095655.

CSIP. (2007). *A common purpose: Recovery in future mental health services*. Joint Position Paper 8. Care Services Improvement Partnership.

Carson, J., & Brewerton, T. (1991). Out of the clinic into the classroom. *Adults Learning, 2*(*9*), 256–257. https://eric.ed.gov/?id=EJ428024.

Carson, J. (2006). *Be your own self-esteem coach*. Whiting and Birch.

Carson, J., Holloway, F., Wolfson, P., & McNary, M. (Eds.) (2008). *Recovery journeys: Stories of coping with mental health problems*. South London and Maudsley NHS Foundation Trust.

Carson, J., McManus, G., & Chander, A. (2010). Recovery: A selective review of the literature. *Mental Health and Social Inclusion, 14*(*1*), 35–44. doi:10.5042/mhsi.2010.0068.

Carson, J., McNary, M., Wolfson, P., & Holloway, F. (2012). The making of a film about recovery. *Mental Health and Social Inclusion, 15*(*2*), 72–78. doi:10.1108/20428301211232478.

Carson, J., & Hurst, R. (2021). Mental health nursing and recovery: The C-CHIME model. *British Journal of Mental Health Nursing, 26*(*3*), 193–196. doi:10.12968/bjmh.2021.0011.

Cordle, H., Fradgley, J., Carson, J., Holloway, F., & Richards, P. (Eds.) (2011). *Psychosis: Stories of recovery and hope*. Quay Publishers.

Davies, S., Wakely, E., Morgan, S., & Carson, J. (Eds.) (2011). *Mental health recovery heroes past and present: A handbook for mental healthcare staff, service users and carers*. Pavilion.

Deegan, P. (1996). Recovery as a journey of the heart. *Psychiatric Rehabilitation Journal, 19*(*3*), 91–97. doi:10.1037/h0101301.

Gyanfi, N., Bhullar, N., Shahid Islam, M., & Usher, K. (2022). Models and frameworks of mental health recovery: A scoping review of the available literature. *Journal of Mental Health*, 1–13. doi:10.1080/09638237.2022.2069713.

Holloway, F. (2008). Recovery: Where does it all come from? In J. Carson, F. Holloway, P. Wolfson, & M. McNary (Eds.), *Recovery journeys: Stories of coping with mental health problems*. South London and Maudsley NHS Foundation Trust.

Hurst, R., & Carson, J. (2021). Be honest: Why did YOU decide to study Psychology? A recent graduate and a professor reflect. *Psychology Teaching Review, 27*(*2*), 22–35.

Khan, N., & Tracy, D. (2022). The challenges and necessity of situating illness narratives of recovery and mental health treatment. *BJPsych Bulletin, 46*(*2*), 77–82. doi:10.1192/bjb.2021.4.

Lomas, T. (2016). *The positive power of negative emotions: How harnessing your darker feelings can help you see a brighter dawn*. Piatkus.

Maudsley NHS. (2010). Recovery and mental illness: Part one [Video]. www.youtube.com/watch?v=purscrXmygc.

McManus, G., Morgan, S., Fradgley, J., & Carson, J. (2009). Recovery heroes: A profile of Gordon McManus. *A Life in the Day, 13*(*4*), 16–19. doi:10.1108/13666282200900037.

McManus, G., & Carson, J. (2012). *From communism to schizophrenia and beyond: One man's long march to recovery.* Whiting and Birch.

Morgan, S., & Carson, J. (2009). The Recovery Group. *Groupwork, 19(1)*, 26–39. doi:10.1921/gpwk.v19i1.662.

Ogilvie, L. & Carson, J. (2023). *Addiction recovery stories: The G-CHIME model.* Emerald.

Perkins, R. (1999). My three psychiatric careers. In P. Barker, P. Campbell, & B. Davidson (Eds), *From the ashes of experience: Reflections on madness, survival, and growth.* Whurr.

Repper, J., & Perkins, R. (2003). *Social inclusion and recovery.* Balliere Tindall.

Rippere, V., & Williams, R. (1985). *Wounded healers: Mental health workers' experiences of depression.* Wiley.

Roberts, G., & Wolfson, P. (2004). The rediscovery of recovery: Open to all. *Advances in Psychiatric Treatment, 10(1)*, 37–48. doi:10.1192/apt.10.1.37.

Slade, M. (2009). The contribution of mental health services to recovery. *Journal of Mental Health, 18(5)*, 367–371. doi:10.3109/09638230903191256.

Ward, M., Chander, A., Robinson, S., Farquharson, Y., & Carson, J. (2010). It's a one man show. *Mental Health Today*, 32–33.

# 3 The CHIME framework

*Robert Hurst*

Connectedness. Hope and optimism. Identity. Meaning in life. Empowerment.

These are the five factors that make up the CHIME framework of recovery (Leamy et al., 2011). But what does each constituent part mean? What do they each bring to recovery? Are they enough? These are the questions that this chapter seeks to address. First, a look at why and how recovery is conceptualised.

## Recovery in academia

With personal recovery being the goal to aspire to for many people with lived experience, how can it be conceptualised? As it transpires, with great difficulty (Davidson, 2020). It is a highly unique process (Ellison et al., 2018), different for each individual (Anthony, 1993). Therefore, the voices of those in recovery have become incredibly important to furthering understanding (Cordle et al., 2011). This includes recovery narratives – first-hand accounts of mental health difficulties that can come in all manner of forms, including the written word (McGranahan et al., 2019). Recovery narratives are generally found to have a positive impact on people with lived experience (Rennick-Egglestone et al., 2019).

Broadly, recovery is conceptualised as a journey, with no set path and no destination (Deegan, 1988). It is also a risk, due to how much challenging work it requires (Ponte, 2020). The highly personal and unique forms that recovery takes means that one single model of recovery cannot be applied - a challenge for mental health services which tend to employ care-pathways and base practice on large amounts of evidence (Slade, 2010).

It could be said that much like recovery itself, our understanding of recovery is a journey rather than a destination. An ultimate model of recovery is impossible. Rather, it is necessary to collaborate with people with lived experience in good faith, to constantly adapt and update our various conceptualisations of recovery to be as universally relevant as possible.

Models and frameworks are by their nature somewhat at odds with personal recovery. But, to paraphrase recovery researcher Mike Slade (Ontario Shores, 2018), their job is to translate lived experiences into the academic and clinical domains, where they can then be applied.

DOI: 10.4324/9781003319405-3

## Development of CHIME

As demonstrated in Chapter 2, the academic study of mental health recovery is nothing new. There is a broad history of conceptualisations and models. For the purposes of this chapter, a sensible place to begin is with notable work by Retta Andresen, Lindsay Oades, and Peter Caputi. After gathering and analysing a broad mixture of recovery narratives and theoretical articles (Andresen et al., 2003), they arrived at a conceptualisation of recovery (Andresen et al., 2011). This involved four component processes: Hope, responsibility, self and identity, meaning and purpose. This work also produced a 5-stage model of recovery, alongside a measure for psychological recovery – the Stages of Recovery Instrument (STORI; Andresen et al., 2006).

Researchers from the United Kingdom conducted their own study, analysing 97 different theoretical conceptualisations of recovery (Leamy et al., 2011). Their findings lined up well with those of Andresen et al., but with the addition of a fifth component process, a social aspect. What they arrived at was a framework involving the five processes mentioned at the start of this chapter, collectively referred to as CHIME. These processes, or dimensions, each have a number of elements associated with them. You can find these detailed in Table 1.1 (adapted from Leamy et al., 2011).

*Table 1.1* Dimensions and elements of CHIME.

| *CHIME dimensions* | *Dimension elements* |
| --- | --- |
| Connectedness | Peer support and support groups |
| | Relationships |
| | Support from others |
| | Being part of the community |
| Hope and optimism about the future | Belief in possibility of recovery |
| | Motivation to change |
| | Hope-inspiring relationships |
| | Positive thinking and valuing success |
| | Having dreams and aspirations |
| Identity | Dimensions of identity |
| | Rebuilding/redefining positive sense of identity |
| | Overcoming stigma |
| Meaning in life | Meaning of mental illness* experiences |
| | Spirituality |
| | Quality of life |
| | Meaningful life and social roles |
| | Meaningful life and social goals |
| | Rebuilding life |
| Empowerment | Personal responsibility |
| | Control over life |
| | Focusing upon strengths |

* Original wording from Leamy et al. (2011). This would perhaps read better as "meaning of lived experiences".

The five dimensions are just that – this is not a stage model. There is no linear progression through, rather it is suggested that these are five processes which underlie personal recovery (Slade et al., 2014). Five foundations which are applied by individuals in their own unique way. The five dimensions are distinct from each other but can interact. For example, if a hypothetical person feels a sense of purpose after inspiring hope in a friend by overcoming stigma to share their mental health story proudly, this scenario incorporates all five dimensions at once.

## The five dimensions

Now the five dimensions of CHIME will be briefly outlined to give readers a sense of what they are, and the ways that they can each impact mental health and recovery.

### Connectedness

No man is an island, entire of itself; every man is a piece of the continent, a part of the main.

(John Donne, 'No Man Is an Island', 1624)

With this quote, poet John Donne accurately sums up the inseparable nature of the individual and the social. The two cannot be disentangled (Grant, 2019). The potentially devastating impact of social isolation was highlighted during the coronavirus pandemic and subsequent lockdowns (Ganesan et al., 2021), with research finding statistical links between loneliness and suicidal ideation (Elbogen et al., 2021). As such it is unsurprising that within CHIME, connectedness is seen as a factor that will increase the likelihood of recovery.

A wealth of studies support this link, from qualitative studies where people with lived experience recognise the importance of having a place in the social world (Kverme et al., 2019), to meta-analyses finding the presence of social relationships to mitigate mortality risks (Holt-Lunstad et al., 2010). The proven efficacy of mental health peer support groups (Lyons et al., 2021) also suggest that social connections with others can play an important role in recovery.

### Hope and optimism

Hope can broadly be defined as a positive, future-oriented, goal-directed mindset (Snyder, 2000). It is a powerful thing. It can affect our mental state in relation to something as everyday as thinking about an exam (Gadosey et al., 2021), and also in times of life-and-death. The Italian writer and chemist Primo Levi witnessed horrors in the concentration camps of the Second World War, yet still hope persisted (Levi, 2017). Indeed, he is quoted as saying "hope is as contagious as despair" (Geras, 2016, p.8).

Hope can be a protective factor, mitigating the risks of post-traumatic stress disorder during times of difficulty (Gallagher et al., 2020). It is seen as an important element of recovery (Van Gestel-Timmermans et al., 2010) due to it giving those with lived experience a sense that things could get better.

### *Identity*

Who are we? When given a diagnosis, does the answer change? These are important questions, especially when considering metal health, where despite years of campaigning and some reduction, stigma is still a very real concern (Bowen & Lovell, 2019). The social weight surrounding words such as "schizophrenia" and the stigma that follows (Valery & Prouteau, 2020) means that a positive identity despite this surely ties in with recovery. As you will read from Andrew Voyce in Chapter 5, moving beyond a self-identity as a "psychiatric patient" was an important milestone in his own recovery journey.

Identity is a multifaceted construct which encompasses the internal and social worlds, sometimes both at once (Brewin, 2023). What identities do we create for ourselves? Which do we share with others? Cruwys et al. (2020) found that recovery group members who identified as "in recovery" had better outcomes, suggesting that by having a strong sense of identity within a social context and feeling "in it together" via their view of self, they would increase chances of better wellbeing.

One way to aid those with lived experience to construct a more positive identity is via a board game (Kerr et al., 2019). While results with a clinical and non-clinical group did not find significant statistical differences between the groups, participants from both populations were able to increase their sense of mastery through playing the game (Kerr et al., 2020), indicating that development of a more positive identity is possible for those on a recovery journey.

### *Meaning in life*

What is it that motivates us on a daily basis? To Viktor Frankl, the answer was meaning (Frankl, 1985). A sometimes-ephemeral construct, meaning can be broadly understood as the experience of finding a sense of purpose in activities or life events at an individual level (King & Hicks, 2021).

For example, this meaning may be found in employment (Ward & King, 2017), with studies finding that participants who see work as a "calling" are more likely to experience better wellbeing (Steger & Dik, 2009). In the literature, not only has meaning in life been found to mediate a reduction in stress (Arslan & Allen, 2022), depression and anxiety (Szcześniak et al., 2022), but also seems to be related to recovery across multiple dimensions - from physical health to happiness (Steger, 2017).

### *Empowerment*

It follows that for a recovery journey to move forward, the individual needs to feel capable of being able to do so – empowered to reach a happy place (Gonot-Schoupinsky et al., 2023). Dell et al. (2021) found in a systematic review of existing systematic reviews of recovery models that one of four key aspects of these models was a sense of autonomy and personal responsibility around the recovery process.

This then translates into practice, too. Researchers in China found that empowerment and personal agency played an important role in recovery from schizophrenia (Ho et al., 2010). Operating within this principle, psychoeducational interventions were found to boost empowerment– in Asia, a programme sought to provide a train-the-trainer system for caregivers. As well as improving empowerment through giving participants the means to teach others, in turn psychological burdens on those participants were reduced (Chiu et al., 2013).

### CHIME in practice

The CHIME framework has been shown to be relatable to those with lived experience of recovery (Voyce, 2020). It has good reliability when applied across cultures – both English speaking (Slade et al., 2012) and non-English speaking (Apostolopoulou et al., 2020; Yung et al., 2021). This makes sense, as CHIME was initially developed with consideration for a diversity of cultures in mind (Leamy et al., 2011). This is important, as different cultures have their own understandings and definitions of mental health recovery (Sofouli, 2021). Different cultures interpret the five dimensions in different ways (Brijnath, 2015), which implies that CHIME is adaptable; a good foundation.

However, not all aspects of recovery narratives map onto the framework, particularly negative experiences in recovery (Stuart et al., 2017). This had led to calls for CHIME to expand, to acknowledge the difficulties that can arise during recovery (van Weeghel et al., 2019).

Despite this criticism, the CHIME framework has been applied clinically. It was used to develop a staff intervention, "REFOCUS", which aimed to give those working in mental health services the skills and knowledge to encourage recovery (Slade et al., 2015b). In an initial trial, quantitative measures showed no change in recovery post-intervention, however service users reported experiencing benefits qualitatively, and staff showed more recovery-oriented behaviour after the intervention (Slade et al., 2015a). An adapted version with an Australian population yielded a small but significant quantitative effect (Meadows et al., 2019).

CHIME can be used as a conversation starter for mental health professionals, facilitating dialogue with service users, and highlighting to staff that what may have seemed mundane aspects of the journey were in fact important to service users (Piat et al., 2017). The framework has also been used as the basis for the development of a mental health recovery questionnaire (Armstrong et al., 2014), allowing practitioners to get a more quantitative sense of how recovery is going for their service users (Lim et al., 2020). It has even been applied in areas outside of mental health recovery, such as in addiction recovery (Ogilvie & Carson, 2021).

### Positive psychology

It is worth pausing to note the parallels (Resnick & Rosenheck, 2006) between recovery and positive psychology (PP). PP is a relatively recent school of thought that has developed in psychology which looks to focus on strengths rather than deficits, wellbeing rather than illness (Seligman & Csikszentmihalyi, 2000).

Andresen et al. (2011) linked PP in with their work, suggesting that it acts as a bridge between lived experience and science. They noted the more scientific approach taken by many positive psychology studies, in an attempt to give strong academic credence to the ideas presented. There is a need for thorough research in order to establish PP as an area to be taken seriously. However, this should not come at the detriment of qualitative, experience-informed research.

Mike Slade, who along with colleagues proposed the CHIME framework, has also made connections between the framework and PP (Slade, 2010). Broadly, CHIME is focused on five strengths that can be developed and harnessed, rather than deficits that need to be reduced. Each of connectedness (Fu & Vong, 2016), hope (Seligman, 2018), identity (Worth, 2020), meaning (Wong, 2020), and empowerment (Hart, 2022) can be seen as PP topics.

Paul Wong's concept of "Positive Psychology 2.0", the idea that while we should certainly focus on positive aspects of psychology we must also remain aware of the negative aspects, supports critiques of CHIME that say it should balance the positive dimensions with an acknowledgement of the negative aspects of recovery (Wong, 2011).

All this to say that not only is CHIME very much in line with the philosophy of PP, but so is this book. We *also* want to focus on strengths, to move away from a medical view of mental health. Our only criticism is the intense focus on scientific, quantitative methods of study. We believe in hearing the voices of those with lived experience.

**Remarkable Lives**

The work of Andresen et al. (2011) and Leamy et al. (2011) was from the top down. They took published, scientific research and looked at that to try and best understand recovery. This was done deliberately, synthesising huge amounts of findings rather than going back and trying to analyse even bigger amounts of primary data. It makes a lot of sense – hundreds of researchers contributed idiographic (or bottom-up, coming directly from lived experience accounts) research to academia, spending many thousands of collective hours gathering, analysing and writing up data. By taking these findings and then analysing them, the best work is brought together, and common themes running through them are found. It is "standing on the shoulders of giants". However, it occurred to us that perhaps it would be worthwhile taking the primary finding of this work, the CHIME framework, and bringing it back down to its idiographic roots. For simplicity and an element of control, we chose to use one curated series of recovery narratives.

As Jerome explained in Chapter 2, Remarkable Lives is a series that began life in 2009 (Sen et al., 2009) as Recovery Heroes, answering Patricia Deegan's call to "try and see the individual [in recovery] as a hero" (Deegan, 1996, p. 95). Inspired by years of hearing remarkable stories of recovery from people he worked with, Jerome wanted to give such individuals an audience. After finding a home in the journal *Mental Health and Social Inclusion*, and changing the name of the series to Remarkable Lives, Jerome got under way.

The papers were co-authored. People with lived experience who were interested in writing for the series would be asked to pen up to 1,000 words, sharing their story. Jerome would then ask them some questions that both professionals and other people with lived experience would hopefully find relevant. These ranged from asking about medication, to experiences with mental health services, to how they would like to be remembered. This was a way of allowing people to tell their stories in their words, while using the Q&A to ground this first-hand narrative in current academic topics. This was done in the intention of avoiding the colonisation of accounts, while also ensuring that there would be some focus on relevant topics for an academic audience. Jerome's main wish was that the stories would serve as an inspiration to others. From personal testimony, I can confirm that this aim has been met.

The writers for Remarkable Lives came from an array of sources. Having just moved to the University of Bolton to become professor of psychology, Jerome found that many of the people he came across who wanted to write their narratives were students.

At the time we embarked upon this research, 36 Remarkable Lives pieces had been written and published. For our first piece (Hurst & Carson, 2021), we cut this number of available accounts almost in half, and focused on the 20 articles authored by students. As well as giving us a fairly even split, this was a way of breaking the set into a demographic. Knowing that all of these people were current/former students gave us a jumping off point in terms of our focus, and meant that we could look to see whether we could glean anything about the impact of education on mental health.

Each account was read thoroughly several times to look for signs of each CHIME dimension. Concurrently, we looked for other emerging themes that came up across the accounts. Several of these were found, including motherhood and education as a positive force. We were able to find evidence of all five CHIME dimensions in each of the 20 accounts. This was a significant indication that CHIME was a useful framework when looking at recovery.

## Creativity in CHIME

A second piece of research looked at the remaining non-student accounts (Hurst et al., 2022). There were 16 in all. These were people of varying backgrounds – there were educators, researchers, activists. Often all three at once.

This time, Robert and Jerome were joined by four other researchers to help ensure that the accounts were being assessed in a reliable way. The emergent themes from the previous analysis were carried over, and each scorer was encouraged to look for new themes, too.

CHIME was once again highly present in these recovery narratives. 15 out of the 16 accounts featured all five dimensions. The one account that could not be mapped onto the framework completely did feature four out of five of the dimensions.

However, the most interesting finding from this analysis was an emerging theme. Each of the researchers noticed that creativity was highly prevalent in the recovery narratives of these 16 individuals. Looking back on the first analysis with this lens, it became clear that all of those accounts also used creativity within their recovery. That they had all been students had prevented us from realising that while education was a big factor in the students' recovery, this was actually a means for them to be creative – as students. We saw coursework instead of creativity.

This led us to wonder whether perhaps CHIME needed to expand to six component processes, with the addition of creativity, to make C-CHIME (Carson & Hurst, 2021). This is what formed the basis of this current research, what led us to wanting to dig deeper into creativity and the impact that it can have on recovery. Just as this chapter bridges recovery and creativity in the context of the book, CHIME was our bridge from recovery to creativity. Examining the 36 accounts in the context of the dimensions of CHIME allowed us to see what else was present in the recovery narratives of the individuals who wrote for Remarkable Lives.

## Conclusion

To readers who were wondering whether the analysis of five stories is enough to produce a framework, here is assurance for you that we were in the first instance influenced by the stories of 36 Remarkable Lives writers. It was through reading their narratives that we first spotted a connection between creativity and recovery. They shaped our initial thinking. We thought some more. Then our five StoryTellers refined our ideas, gave us examples and context and insights we did not have. There have been further Remarkable Lives published since (e.g. Stacey & Hurst, 2022), which now ask questions specifically about creativity. The answers so far have supported our line of thinking.

Before we examine the research that we carried out, we must first attempt to understand what creativity is.

## References

Andresen, R., Caputi, P., & Oades, L. (2006). Stages of recovery instrument: Development of a measure of recovery from serious mental illness. *Australian & New Zealand Journal of Psychiatry*, *40*(*11–12*), 972–980. doi:10.1080/j.1440-1614.2006.01921.x.

Andresen, R., Oades, L. G., & Caputi, P. (2011). *Psychological recovery: Beyond mental illness*. John Wiley & Sons.

Andresen, R., Oades, L., & Caputi, P. (2003). The experience of recovery from schizophrenia: Towards an empirically validated stage model. *Australian & New Zealand Journal of Psychiatry*, *37*(*5*), 586–594. doi:10.1046%2Fj.1440-1614.2003.01234.x.

Anthony, W. A. (1993). Recovery from mental illness: The guiding vision of the mental health service system in the 1990s. *Psychosocial Rehabilitation Journal*, *16*(*4*), 11–23. doi:10.1037/h0095655.

Apostolopoulou, A., Stylianidis, S., Issari, P., Chondros, P., Alexiadou, A., Belekou, P., Giannou, C., Karali, K., Foi, V., & Tzaferou, F. (2020). Experiences of recovery in EPAPSY's community residential facilities and the five CHIME concepts: A qualitative inquiry. *Frontiers in Psychiatry*, *11*, 24. doi:10.3389/fpsyt.2020.00024.

Armstrong, N. P., Cohen, A. N., Hellemann, G., Reist, C., & Young, A. S. (2014). Validating a brief version of the mental health recovery measure for individuals with schizophrenia. *Psychiatric Services, 65*(*9*), 1154–1159. doi:10.1176/appi.ps.201300215.

Arslan, G., & Allen, K. A. (2022). Exploring the association between coronavirus stress, meaning in life, psychological flexibility, and subjective well-being. *Psychology, Health & Medicine, 27*(*4*), 803–814. doi:10.1080/13548506.2021.1876892.

Bowen, M., & Lovell, A. (2019). Stigma: The representation of mental health in UK newspaper Twitter feeds. *Journal of Mental Health, 30*(*4*), 424–430. doi:10.1080/09638237.2019.1608937.

Brewin, C. R. (2023). Identity – A critical but neglected construct in cognitive-behaviour therapy. *Journal of Behavior Therapy and Experimental Psychiatry, 78*, 101808. doi:10.1016/j.jbtep.2022.101808.

Brijnath, B. (2015). Applying the CHIME recovery framework in two culturally diverse Australian communities: Qualitative results. *International Journal of Social Psychiatry, 61*(*7*), 660–667. doi:10.1177%2F0020764015573084.

Carson, J., & Hurst, R. (2021). Mental health nursing and recovery: The C-CHIME model. *British Journal of Mental Health Nursing, 10*(*2*), 1–3. doi:10.12968.bjmh.2021.0011.

Chiu, M. Y., Wei, G. F., Lee, S., Choovanichvong, S., & Wong, F. H. (2013). Empowering caregivers: Impact analysis of FamilyLink Education Programme (FLEP) in Hong Kong, Taipei and Bangkok. *International Journal of Social Psychiatry, 59*(*1*), 28–39. doi:10.1177/0020764011423171.

Cordle, H., Fradgley, J., Carson, J., Holloway, F., & Richards, P. (Eds.) (2011). *Psychosis: Stories of recovery and hope.* Quay Books.

Cruwys, T., Stewart, B., Buckley, L., Gumley, J., & Scholz, B. (2020). The recovery model in chronic mental health: A community-based investigation of social identity processes. *Psychiatry Research, 291*, 113241. doi:10.1016/j.psychres.2020.113241.

Davidson, L. (2020). What is recovery? In K. Ponte (Ed.), *For like minds: Mental illness recovery insights* (pp. 77–81). Real MH Works.

Deegan, P. (1996). Recovery as a journey of the heart. *Psychiatric Rehabilitation Journal, 19*(*3*), 91–97. doi:10.1037/h0101301.

Deegan, P. E. (1988). Recovery: The lived experience of rehabilitation. *Psychosocial Rehabilitation Journal, 11*(*4*), 11–19. doi:10.1037/h0099565.

Dell, N. A., Long, C., & Mancini, M. A. (2021). Models of mental health recovery: An overview of systematic reviews and qualitative meta-syntheses. *Psychiatric Rehabilitation Journal, 44*(*3*), 238. doi:10.1037/prj0000444.

Donne, J. (1839). *The works of John Donne.* John W. Parker.

Elbogen, E. B., Lanier, M., Blakey, S. M., Wagner, H. R., & Tsai, J. (2021). Suicidal ideation and thoughts of self-harm during the COVID-19 pandemic: The role of COVID-19-related stress, social isolation, and financial strain. *Depression and Anxiety, 38*(*7*), 739–748. doi:10.1002/da.23162.

Ellison, M. L., Belanger, L. K., Niles, B. L., Evans, L. C., & Bauer, M. S. (2018). Explication and definition of mental health recovery: A systematic review. *Administration and Policy in Mental Health and Mental Health Services Research, 45*(*1*), 91–102. doi:10.1007/s10488-016-0767-9.

Frankl, V. E. (1985). *Man's search for meaning.* Simon & Schuster.

Fu, M., & Vong, S. (2016). Social connectedness can lead to happiness: Positive psychology and Asian Americans. In E. C. Chang, C. A. Downey, J. K. Hirsch, & N. J. Lin (Eds.), *Positive psychology in racial and ethnic groups: Theory, research, and practice* (pp. 217–233). American Psychological Association. doi:10.1037/14799-011.

Gadosey, C. K., Schnettler, T., Scheunemann, A., Fries, S., & Grunschel, C. (2021). The intraindividual co-occurrence of anxiety and hope in procrastination episodes during exam preparations: An experience sampling study. *Learning and Individual Differences*, *88*, 102013. doi:10.1016/j.lindif.2021.102013.

Gallagher, M. W., Long, L. J., & Phillips, C. A. (2020). Hope, optimism, self-efficacy, and posttraumatic stress disorder: A meta-analytic review of the protective effects of positive expectancies. *Journal of Clinical Psychology*, *76*(*3*), 329–355. doi:10.1002/jclp.22882.

Ganesan, B., Al-Jumaily, A., Fong, K. N., Prasad, P., Meena, S. K., & Tong, R. K. Y. (2021). Impact of coronavirus disease 2019 (COVID-19) outbreak quarantine, isolation, and lockdown policies on mental health and suicide. *Frontiers in Psychiatry*, *12*, 565190. doi:10.3389/fpsyt.2021.565190.

Geras, N. (2016). Hope, shame, and resentment: Primo Levi and Jean Améry. In M. Vuohelainen & A. Chapman (Eds.), *Interpreting Primo Levi* (pp. 7–20). Palgrave Macmillan. doi:10.1057/9781137435576_2.

Gonot-Schoupinsky, F., Weeks, M., & Carson, J. (2023). "You can end up in a happy place" (Voyce): A role for positive autoethnography. *Mental Health and Social Inclusion*, *27*(*4*), 380–391. doi:10.1108/MHSI-02-2023-0021.

Grant, A. (2019). Dare to be a wolf: Embracing autoethnography in nurse educational research. *Nurse Education Today*, *82*, 88–92. doi:10.1016/j.nedt.2019.07.006.

Hart, J. (2022). Positive Psychology: One way to empower patients during the pandemic. *Integrative and Complementary Therapies*, *28*(*1*), 28–30. doi:10.1089/ict.2021.29001.jha.

Ho, W. W., Chiu, M. Y., Lo, W. T., & Yiu, M. G. (2010). Recovery components as determinants of the health-related quality of life among patients with schizophrenia: Structural equation modelling analysis. *Australian & New Zealand Journal of Psychiatry*, *44*(*1*), 71–84. doi:10.3109/00048670903393654.

Holt-Lunstad, J., Smith, T. B., & Layton, J. B. (2010). Social relationships and mortality risk: A meta-analytic review. *PLoS Medicine*, *7*(*7*), e1000316. doi:10.1371/journal.pmed.1000316.

Hurst, R., & Carson, J. (2021). For whom the bell CHIMEs: A synthesis of remarkable student lives. *Mental Health and Social Inclusion*, *25*(*2*), 195–207. doi:10.1108/MHSI-10-2020-0071.

Hurst, R., Carson, J., Shahama, A., Kay, H., Nabb, C., & Prescott, J. (2022). Remarkable recoveries: An interpretation of recovery narratives using the CHIME model. *Mental Health and Social Inclusion*, *26*(*2*), 175–190. doi:10.1108/MHSI-01-2022-0001.

Kerr, D. J., Deane, F. P., & Crowe, T. P. (2019). Narrative identity reconstruction as adaptive growth during mental health recovery: A narrative coaching boardgame approach. *Frontiers in Psychology*, *10*, 994. doi:10.3389/fpsyg.2019.00994.

Kerr, D. J., Deane, F. P., & Crowe, T. P. (2020). Pilot study of a serious board game intervention to facilitate narrative identity reconstruction in mental health recovery. *Health Psychology Open*, *7*(*1*), 2055102920905628. doi:10.1177/2055102920905628.

King, L. A., & Hicks, J. A. (2021). The science of meaning in life. *Annual Review of Psychology*, *72*, 561–584. doi:10.1146/annurev-psych-072420-122921.

Kverme, B., Natvik, E., Veseth, M., & Moltu, C. (2019). Moving toward connectedness–a qualitative study of recovery processes for people with borderline personality disorder. *Frontiers in Psychology*, *10*, 430. doi:10.3389/fpsyg.2019.00430.

Leamy, M., Bird, V., Le Boutillier, C., Williams, J., & Slade, M. (2011). Conceptual framework for personal recovery in mental health: Systematic review and narrative synthesis. *The British Journal of Psychiatry*, *199*(*6*), 445–452. doi:10.1192/bjp.bp.110.083733.

Levi, P. (2017). *The drowned and the saved.* Simon & Schuster.

Lim, M., Xie, H., Li, Z., Tan, B. L., & Lee, J. (2020). Using the CHIME Personal Recovery Framework to evaluate the validity of the MHRM-10 in individuals with psychosis. *Psychiatric Quarterly, 91(3),* 793–805. doi:10.1007/s11126-020-09737-2.

Lyons, N., Cooper, C., & Lloyd-Evans, B. (2021). A systematic review and meta-analysis of group peer support interventions for people experiencing mental health conditions. *BMC Psychiatry, 21(1),* 1–17. doi:10.1186/s12888-021-03321-z.

McGranahan, R., Rennick-Egglestone, S., Ramsay, A., Llewellyn-Beardsley, J., Bradstreet, S., Callard, F., Priebe, S., & Slade, M. (2019). Curation of mental health recovery narrative collections: Systematic review and qualitative synthesis. *JMIR Mental Health, 6(10),* e14233. doi:10.2196/14233.

Meadows, G., Brophy, L., Shawyer, F., Enticott, J. C., Fossey, E., Thornton, C. D., Weller, P. J., Wilson-Evered, E., Edan, V., & Slade, M. (2019). REFOCUS-PULSAR recovery-oriented practice training in specialist mental health care: A stepped-wedge cluster randomised controlled trial. *The Lancet Psychiatry, 6(2),* 103–114. doi:10.1016/S2215-0366(18)30429-2.

Ogilvie, L., & Carson, J. (2021). Addiction recovery stories: Jerome Carson in conversation with Lisa Ogilvie. *Advances in Dual Diagnosis, 15(2),* 73–78. doi:10.1108/ADD-12-2021-0015.

Ontario Shores. (2018). #MindVine podcast episode 47 – Dr. Mike Slade [Video]. www.youtube.com/watch?v=5GdduBDctfk

Piat, M., Seida, K., & Sabetti, J. (2017). Understanding everyday life and mental health recovery through CHIME. *Mental Health and Social Inclusion, 21(5),* 271–279. doi:10.1108/MHSI-08-2017-0034.

Ponte, K. (2020). A risk too big not to take: A story of recovery. *Psychiatric Services, 71(5),* 516–517. doi:10.1176/appi.ps.71401.

Rennick-Egglestone, S., Morgan, K., Llewellyn-Beardsley, J., Ramsay, A., McGranahan, R., Gillard, S., … & Slade, M. (2019). Mental health recovery narratives and their impact on recipients: Systematic review and narrative synthesis. *The Canadian Journal of Psychiatry, 64(10),* 669–679. doi:10.1177/0706743719846108.

Resnick, S. G., & Rosenheck, R. A. (2006). Recovery and positive psychology: Parallel themes and potential synergies. *Psychiatric Services, 57(1),* 120–122. doi:10.1176/appi.ps.57.1.120.

Seligman, M. E. (2018). *The hope circuit: A psychologist's journey from helplessness to optimism.* Hachette UK.

Seligman, M. E., & Csikszentmihalyi, M. (2000). Positive psychology: An introduction. *American Psychologist, 55(1),* 5–14. doi:10.1037//0003-066X.55.1.5.

Sen, D., Morgan, S., & Carson, J. (2009). Recovery heroes - A profile of Dolly Sen. *A Life in the Day, 13(2),* 6–8. doi:10.1108/13666282200900013.

Slade, M. (2010). Mental illness and well-being: The central importance of positive psychology and recovery approaches. *BMC Health Services Research, 10(1),* 1–14. doi:10.1186/1472-6963-10-26.

Slade, M., Amering, M., Farkas, M., Hamilton, B., O'Hagan, M., Panther, G., Perkins, R., Shepherd, G., Tse, S., & Whitley, R. (2014). Uses and abuses of recovery: Implementing recovery-oriented practices in mental health systems. *World Psychiatry, 13(1),* 12–20. doi:10.1002/wps.20084.

Slade, M., Bird, V., Clarke, E., Le Boutillier, C., McCrone, P., Macpherson, R., Pesola, F., Wallace, G., Williams, J., & Leamy, M. (2015a). Supporting recovery in patients with psychosis through care by community-based adult mental health teams (REFOCUS): A multisite, cluster, randomised, controlled trial. *The Lancet Psychiatry*, *2*(*6*), 503–514. doi:10.1016/S2215-0366(15)00086-3.

Slade, M., Bird, V., Le Boutillier, C., Farkas, M., Grey, B., Larsen, J., Leamy, M., Oades, L., & Williams, J. (2015b). Development of the REFOCUS intervention to increase mental health team support for personal recovery. *The British Journal of Psychiatry*, *207*(*6*), 544–550. doi:10.1192/bjp.bp.114.155978.

Slade, M., Leamy, M., Bacon, F., Janosik, M., Le Boutillier, C., Williams, J., & Bird, V. (2012). International differences in understanding recovery: Systematic review. *Epidemiology and Psychiatric Sciences*, *21*(4), 353–364. doi:10.1017/S2045796012000133.

Snyder, C. R. (2000). *Handbook of hope*. Academic Press. doi:10.1016/B978-012654050-5/50003-8.

Sofouli, E. (2021). Cross-cultural conceptualization and implementation of recovery in mental health: A literature review. *Mental Health and Social Inclusion*, *25*(*1*), 32–40. doi:10.1108/MHSI-08-2020-0057.

Stacey, K., & Hurst, R. (2022). Remarkable lives: Khia Stacey in conversation with Robert Hurst. *Mental Health and Social Inclusion*, *26*(*4*), 418–424. doi:10.1108/MHSI-03-2022-0015.

Steger, M. F. (2017). Meaning in life and wellbeing. In M. Slade, L. Oades & A. Jarden (Eds.), *Wellbeing, recovery and mental health* (pp. 75–85). Cambridge University Press. doi:10.1017/9781316339275.008.

Steger, M. F., & Dik, B. J. (2009). If one is looking for meaning in life, does it help to find meaning in work? *Applied Psychology: Health and Well-Being*, *1*(*3*), 303–320. doi:10.1111/j.1758-0854.2009.01018.x.

Stuart, S. R., Tansey, L., & Quayle, E. (2017). What we talk about when we talk about recovery: A systematic review and best-fit framework synthesis of qualitative literature. *Journal of Mental Health*, *26*(*3*), 291–304. doi:10.1080/09638237.2016.1222056.

Szcześniak, M., Falewicz, A., Strochalska, K., & Rybarski, R. (2022). Anxiety and depression in a non-clinical sample of young polish adults: Presence of meaning in life as a mediator. *International Journal of Environmental Research and Public Health*, *19*(*10*), 6065. doi:10.3390/ijerph19106065.

Valery, K. M., & Prouteau, A. (2020). Schizophrenia stigma in mental health professionals and associated factors: A systematic review. *Psychiatry Research*, *290*, 113068. doi:10.1016/j.psychres.2020.113068.

Van Gestel-Timmermans, H., Van Den Bogaard, J., Brouwers, E., Herth, K., & Van Nieuwenhuizen, C. (2010). Hope as a determinant of mental health recovery: A psychometric evaluation of the Herth Hope Index-Dutch version. *Scandinavian Journal of Caring Sciences*, *24*, 67–74. doi:10.1111/j.1471-6712.2009.00758.x.

van Weeghel, J., van Zelst, C., Boertien, D., & Hasson-Ohayon, I. (2019). Conceptualizations, assessments, and implications of personal recovery in mental illness: A scoping review of systematic reviews and meta-analyses. *Psychiatric Rehabilitation Journal*, *42*(2), 169–181. doi:10.1037/prj0000356.

Voyce, A. (2020). Two narratives: Recovery journeys in mental health. *Mental Health and Social Inclusion*, *24*(2), 105–110. doi:10.1108/MHSI-03-2020-0011.

Ward, S. J., & King, L. A. (2017). Work and the good life: How work contributes to meaning in life. *Research in Organizational Behavior*, *37*, 59–82. doi:10.1016/j.riob.2017.10.001.

Wong, P. T. (2011). Positive psychology 2.0: Towards a balanced interactive model of the good life. *Canadian Psychology/Psychologie Canadienne*, *52*(2), 69–81. doi:10.1037/a0022511.

Wong, P. T. (2020). Existential positive psychology and integrative meaning therapy. *International Review of Psychiatry*, *32*(7–8), 565–578. doi:10.1080/09540261.2020.1814703.

Worth, P. (2020). The potential use of 'positive psychology interventions' as a means of affecting individual senses of identity and coping capacity impacted by 4IR job and employment changes. *International Review of Psychiatry*, *32*(7–8), 606–615. doi:10.1080/09540261.2020.1814222.

Yung, J. Y., Wong, V., Ho, G. W., & Molassiotis, A. (2021). Understanding the experiences of hikikomori through the lens of the CHIME framework: Connectedness, hope and optimism, identity, meaning in life, and empowerment; systematic review. *BMC Psychology*, *9*(1), 1–30. doi:10.1186/s40359-021-00605-7.

# 4 Creativity and recovery

*Robert Hurst*

200,000 years ago, in what would later be called Tibet, there are children playing. One is 7 years old, the other 12. They are making patterns in the mud using their handprints. Art. One can only assume they expect their creation to be ephemeral, to be washed away by the elements. But in fact it fossilized, creating humanity's oldest remnant of art. It is agreed to be an example of parietal art because it is intentional. Not because it is beautiful, but because "care appears to have been taken with the composition" (Zhang et al., 2021, p. 2510).

These children left an imprint of themselves that echoed through the centuries, a marker of their existence and intelligence. Their art is now used as evidence for *Homo sapiens* at the time that they lived. Here, historians see creativity as a marker of humanity. That is how important it is, what a big part of *us* it is. So how have academics explained and conceptualised this phenomenon?

## Creativity conceptualisations

As with recovery, creativity has many definitions (Ford & Harris, 1992). What is sometimes referred to as the "standard version" (Runco & Jaeger, 2012), is that creativity requires an output that is original (Treffert, 1989) and of value (Andreasen, 2006). Csikszentmihalyi (1990) takes this further, positing that these original works must be seen as noteworthy within their domain (area of activity) by the field (domain experts, gatekeepers such as gallery curators and publishers). By this definition, he notes that people not recognised within their lifetimes only become creative many years after their death when their work is positively appraised. These appear to be odd *psychological* definitions of creativity, as they do not describe creativity as an internal force happening within a mind, but as something based on how creative *outputs* are viewed by others and society.

Implying that a painter only becomes creative after they have died is absurd (Weisberg, 2015), as it is not focused on when that painter was in a creative psychological state, but on when others have passed the appropriate judgement on the works that were created. By this definition, Vincent van Gogh was not creative until many years after his death. A dead man sitting with his sunflowers. If somebody writes a small poem, which they keep to themselves – this is not seen as

DOI: 10.4324/9781003319405-4

creative. Though creativity can happen at a societal level or within groups (Edgell & Lee, 2023), it can also be an entirely solitary act.

The implication that there are domain rules that need to be followed for something to be creative, that creativity is about "solving problems" in the "real world" (Mumford & England, 2022), also appears to be something of a contradiction. "Thinking outside of the box" is a phrase for when somebody comes up with an *unexpected* solution – when they *break* the domain rules. Indeed, such divergent thinking has been found to predict creativity (Shaw, 2023).

This fuelled a call for the definition to be amended to novel works that have been created intentionally (Weisberg, 2006). Yet, this *also* ignores the psychological process behind the final output. The idea that creativity needs to be novel works to dehumanise those doing the creating, with scholars reducing creativity to "average novelty values" (Harrington, 2018, p. 120) and other such phrases. Creativity scholars seem to cling to the "novel" requirement as it is an extension of the eminence that the "usefulness" element of the definition appears to be seeking. This allows for work to be more scientifically measurable, with scales from big name psychologists seemingly reflecting this (Carson et al., 2005), with bizarre items such as "I have been asked to prepare food for celebrities or dignitaries" within a scale claiming to measure creativity. Yet these works do not, to my mind, address the central issue of who decides *what* is novel.

Take this scenario. Two people begin to paint a picture. They live on opposite sides of the world from one another, and exist within entirely different cultural contexts. Neither has ever met the other, and the only thing that connects them is that they both sit before an easel with a brush and some paint. Both paint the exact same picture in terms of subject, composition, colour choices – whether by chance or because of similar influences. Are these people, when applying paint to canvas, still both creative? The paintings are not, in the true sense, novel. But to each of them, their own painting *is* novel. And yet to a hypothetical, omniscient researcher, neither painting is novel, and so neither person was creative. This seems an absurdity. An injustice.

This highlights an issue within psychological study of creativity, whereby writers seem to confuse "creativity" with "talent" or "art". As one art critic pointed out "creativity is called for and admired in countless other areas of life beyond art" (Dutton, 2006). Many psychology scholars appear to have been distracted by the end-product, the creation, rather than the act of creativity itself (Walia, 2019).

While there is much critique to be made of such fixations on novelty and usefulness, I will attempt to make a clear distinction as to what I consider to be a psychological concept of creativity before we move forward. A more process-based view of creativity conceptualises it as a complicated journey from an idea to a product (Mumford & Gustafson, 1988). It is an act, whereby a person creates something – whether that be a physical object or a mental construct (Vygotsky, 2004). The act does not necessarily need to be intentional, and may not have a specific goal in mind, but it is future-oriented (Glăveanu & Beghetto, 2021). In this way parallels could be drawn to personal recovery, with creativity as a chaotic (Rothouse, 2023) and non-linear process (Sawyer, 2021) with no particular endpoint but rather a forward-moving momentum.

## Big-C and little-c

Beyond an overarching definition, researchers have suggested various kinds of creativity. The most useful for our purposes is "big-C" and "little-c" creativity. This differentiates between eminent people in the arts and sciences (Kaufman & Sternberg, 2010) and creativity expressed by everybody (Andreasen & Ramchandran, 2012). This perhaps balances the scales between the novelty/utility camp and the process camp, by giving them both space within a conceptualisation of creativity. We are all capable of creativity – some creative output is more socially valued, but the thinking processes used in creativity are the same for all of us (Weisberg, 2006).

This C/creativity concept has been criticised for being a false dichotomy (Runco, 2014), and is perhaps better viewed as two ends of a continuum (Kaufman & Sternberg, 2010). By acknowledging everyday creativity, it avoids disenfranchising people from their creativity by telling them that they must make a novel and useful contribution to a domain. Rather than usefulness, everyday creativity focuses on meaningfulness as a driver of creation (Richards, 2018). It liberates creativity from the eminent, allowing it to be studied as something that anybody can do, something that everybody does do (Ilha Villanova & Pina e Cunha, 2021) – it sees creativity as a way of life (Richards, 2010).

I would argue that the Big-C Creativity, which relies of external judgements, is a more social concept such as "talent", "genius", or "artisticness". Little-c creativity appears to be much more psychologically grounded and accessible to anyone, which surely is what creativity is – after all, as highlighted in the introduction to this chapter, it appears that the urge to create is as old as humanity itself. Art and the ability to produce art has an important place in psychological literature, but if creativity is the universal experience that others and I claim, then it needs to be distinguished and not gatekept nor colonised by a need for value judgements.

The founder of person-centred therapy, Carl Rogers, would appear to agree with this assessment. He saw creativity as "the emergence in action of a novel relational product, growing out of the uniqueness of the individual on the one hand and the materials, events, people, or circumstances of his life on the other" (Rogers, 1967, p. 350). Here, creativity is an internal process, by which something (either psychological or physical) unique to the individual is created, which may at a later date be shared with others. The process can be conscious or intuitive (Hardman, 2021). The creation is connected to and therefore an extension of the self. This is the definition from which I am approaching this work, as it seems to be the most in line with the principles of personal recovery.

With that in mind, the remainder of the chapter will explore the existing literature on how creativity impacts wellbeing and recovery.

## Creativity and wellbeing

Psychology has historically tended to have a fixation with creativity in the context of the perceived link between creativity and unwellness – the so-called phenomenon of the "mad genius" (Pickover, 1998). This is often based on anachronistic diagnoses given to long-dead historical figures such as Vincent van Gogh (Nettle, 2001) and Virginia Woolf (Storr, 1993).

Given the "standard" definition of creativity as requiring an element of utility in the creative product, it is ironic that such texts do not pause to critically examine how useful this "mad genius" hypothesis actually is to the field. The discourse can be reduced to a chicken/egg situation, where the link between illness and creativity is strong and interesting but brings forth no discussion of practical implications for mental health. Rather, the focus is more often on promoting more "extraordinary creativity" (Andreasen, 2006). Some attempts at understanding "genius" in a mental health context have been somewhat wrong-headed, with one claiming that just the right level of mental unwellness will provide a person with enough time in solitude such as to improve their thinking and ideas (Pickering, 1974). That this notion requires the unwell person to be financially secure enough to withdraw from society and cultivate their genius is not acknowledged.

For the present work, such lines of thought are irrelevant and potentially harmful. Fortunately, much contemporary literature has attempted to understand what wellbeing benefits creativity may hold.

Contrary to the common suggestion of "mad geniuses", creativity seems to be more prevalent in people who are well-balanced mentally, as often mental unwellness actually prohibits creativity (Sawyer, 2011). Creativity has been found to have a positive correlation with positive affect (Amabile et al., 2005), though which causes which is unclear.

Studies of non-clinical populations have shown a link between creativity and wellbeing. Arnout and Almoied (2021) studied a sample of over 600 counsellors, finding that wellbeing was a strong factor associated with creativity. Encouraging creativity has been proposed as a way of increasing wellbeing in school (Henriksen & Shack, 2020) and university (Peyvastegar, 2010) students. Another study with a mixed sample of both students and working adults found not only a link between the two concepts, but that a creativity priming task boosted the wellbeing scores of participants (Tan et al., 2021).

Doing creative activities, such as improvised dance (Łucznik et al., 2021) and quilting (Burt & Atkinson, 2012), which involve being in a state of flow have also been empirically linked with increased wellbeing. Indeed, if we consider a state of flow (Csikszentmihalyi, 1990) to be an indicator of creativity at work (Schutte & Malouff, 2020) then there is a breadth of literature linking flow positively with wellbeing in various contexts (Fritz & Avsec, 2007; Vyas, 2021).

Coming from a different angle, Mulatti and Treccani (2023) found evidence suggesting that creativity could be triggered by a perceived lack of control – that perhaps our "divergent thinking" in creative ways acts as a kind of defence mechanism to protect our wellbeing.

When thinking about short term goals, it was found that participants who engaged in a creative task felt less worried than a control group who did no creative activity (Reiter et al., 2023) – something about being around and engaging in this creativity made their upcoming plans seem less anxiety-inducing. This change in mindset was also found by Reid-Wisdom and Perera-Delcourt (2022) when investigating the effects of partaking in improvisation. These internal changes then had positives external consequences.

The literature suggests that being actively engaged in creativity can have myriad general positive effects on psychological wellbeing. However, other research has focused more specifically on the impact of creativity for those on a recovery journey.

## Creativity and recovery

Gillam (2018) proposed a new model of creative mental health care, not just for the wellbeing of service users but for the wellbeing of staff too. This is further indication that creativity can have benefits for everybody. However, it has also been shown to be a powerful tool for helping specifically those who are in mental health recovery – a "springboard back to life" (Salomon-Gimmon, 2023).

In the context of recovery, much creativity-related research has focused on various forms of art therapy. For example, groups where service users make visual art have been shown to encourage recovery (Ryan et al., 2021). In a study of Fijian service users, Fenner et al. (2022) found that being in an art group where paints and tactile materials were used enhanced participants' experience of recovery. The artmaking increased their sense of social belonging and identity. Another study found that creating art was a form of exploration, and that when looking back on previous creations, participants were able to explain how the creative process had helped them to make sense of themselves and the world (Van Lith, 2014).

Nitzan and Orkibi (2022) found that through art-based groups, people in recovery could develop their creative self-efficacy, which in turn boosted their overall self-efficacy. Interestingly, the study found that the interventions delivered by creative therapists were more effective than those delivered by other helping professionals, suggesting that the creative aspect was key to the benefits.

Inclusion and connectedness are key themes highlighted by various studies into art-based interventions (Stewart et al., 2019; Williams et al., 2020). Given that the CHIME framework highlights this as one of five key dimensions for recovery, this suggests the potential power of creativity in healing. Indeed, a systematic review by Goodman-Casanova et al. (2023) found that participation in community art groups could lead to benefits in all five dimensions of the CHIME framework to different degrees. Alongside the connectedness generated by partaking in art groups, there is an opportunity to express emotions and parts of the self within these social settings (Jay et al., 2023).

Music-making is another form of applied creativity with a strong empirical base for aiding recovery (Silverman, 2019). For example, one study found that participants of drumming groups felt the benefits of the creative process in their recovery – particularly through a felt sense of community, feeling in-touch with natural rhythms, and performing a physical act (Perkins et al., 2016). Music-making has been mapped onto the CHIME framework, implying that this form of creativity is incredibly useful in aiding recovery journeys across the five dimensions (Damsgaard & Jensen, 2021).

In a pilot study of a remote drama therapy for people with serious mental health diagnoses, Cheung et al. (2022) found no significant quantitative differences, but the qualitative data showed themes of participants processing things that they had been through and adapting their sense of self through the drama activities. This highlights that benefits of creativity are sometimes perhaps too ephemeral and nuanced for quantitative measures to capture.

Another form of creative intervention is creative writing – in a sample of people who had experienced early psychosis, Romm et al. (2022) found that creative writing in group interventions imbued a sense of mastery into participants – it left them feeling a sense of control around how they could express themselves creatively, which maps onto the empowerment domain of CHIME.

A scoping study by Ludowyke et al. (2023) suggested that as well as various art groups, individuals on a recovery journey also found benefits from engaging in their own, personal, everyday creativities outside of intervention settings. Because of this, they suggested that community buildings and institutions should consider the importance of providing space for individuals to be able to express and conduct their everyday creative acts. This was echoed by Hansen et al. (2023), who found that individuals with serious mental health diagnoses saw improvements in their daily living when engaging with their creativity, and that this creativity provided a sense of purpose not unlike that of being in work. When it is considered that some mental health conditions are impactful enough that people are unable to work (Boardman & Rinaldi, 2021), and that work provides a sense of meaning (Ward & King, 2017), this finding seems impactful and strengthens the call for further work into empowering people to engage with their everyday creativity.

It is clear from the literature that being immersed in creative activities and creative social settings provides benefits to those in recovery. But what if somebody is at a stage of their recovery journey where they feel unable to be creative?

**Experiencing creativity**

Something evident through scouring the literature is that it is not only being engaged in a personal creative process that can be beneficial – immersing oneself in creative works by others can also lead to positive outcomes. Throughout history, those with wealth have sought to surround themselves with art – from the Pope hiring Michaelangelo to paint the Sistine Chapel, to the rich and the wealthy collecting and sponsoring artistic works, it is clear that something draws us to beautiful things beyond mere prestige.

The possible therapeutic value of experiencing the creativity of others is shown in a recent trial in Brussels, where psychiatrists offered "museum prescriptions" as a way to reduce depression, anxiety, and stress (Rankin, 2022). Academic literature supports this idea.

Slanzi et al. (2023) found that individuals with serious mental health diagnoses had similar if not stronger desires to participate in The Arts (such as going to the theatre), and that doing so was associated positively with quality of life and recovery. Yet, people with diagnoses were less likely to actively participate in these.

More specifically, reading fictional stories can be therapeutic (Wang et al., 2020), and has been harnessed in a form of therapy called creative bibliotherapy (Glavin & Montgomery, 2017). Tribe et al. (2021) interviewed six Harry Potter fans, and in the analysis found that the stories had had a profound, positive effect in participants' recovery journeys. Participants were able to emotionally identify with characters in the books, but also make connections with other fans of the series, aiding their connectedness and social inclusion. This indicates that creativity is an important aspect of recovery not only when a person is themselves creating, but also when they are engaging with the creations of somebody else.

The same appears to be true of film – researchers found that using the film "Spiderman: Into The Spider-Verse" was successful in better engaging clients in a family therapy context (Smedley & Croffie, 2023). This suggests that media (such as films and books) can act as an emotional or narrative bridge between individuals, even when it has been created by a complete stranger to them.

This demonstrates that perhaps the recovery-boosting power of creativity lies not just in the process of oneself being creative, but in engaging with the creative works of others. One theory that could explain this is narrative creativity. Fletcher et al. (2023) expanded existing theories of narrative creativity to consider that engaging in narrative worlds could strengthen creativity in elementary school children – that this creativity within somebody else's created world could be nourishing (Fletcher & Benveniste, 2022). While they look at this in the context of training minds to be more creative, it follows logically that this narrative creativity and being involved with it could explain the literature that says that experiencing the creativity of others has psychological benefits – it's a means by which individuals can flex their narrative creativity in a slightly more passive and accessible way than their own divergent or convergent creativity.

## Creative space

As well as experiencing others' creativity, research also demonstrates that being immersed in a creative environment can also aid recovery. This might be an environment that is already centred around creativity, such as an art gallery (Colbert et al., 2013), or a space that is purposely curated to be creative as a means of facilitating recovery (De Ruysscher et al., 2022). Sui et al. (2023) found through qualitative research that intentionally making a space that contains art and other visually engaging stimuli could benefit the recovery work undertaken there. This speaks to the possible benefits of aesthetics, of being around things that are beautiful.

A point worth noting here is that for people with serious mental health difficulties, the nature of their condition could affect their ability to engage on an aesthetic level. Pino et al. (2023) conducted an eye-tracking experiment with people who had a diagnosis of schizophrenia, and found that they experienced the aesthetics of visual stimuli in a different way to the non-diagnosed control group. They do not experience aesthetics in a *worse* way, rather in a *different* way. This is not to say that aesthetic or creative forms of intervention should not be offered to people with a schizophrenia diagnosis, but to remain mindful that they may engage with this differently from other individuals, depending on the way that they are affected cognitively. Indeed, this simply further highlights the reasons to avoid placing value judgements upon creativity – it will look different to everybody!

Jensen (2018) conducted a piece of research that involved people on recovery journeys visiting a series of museums in Copenhagen as both "viewers" and "makers" of arts. After a guided tour of the museum, participants took part in a relevant workshop. Qualitative inquiry found this to be an overall successful approach – participants found a great deal of meaning and empowerment from visiting these creative spaces and being able to then create within them themselves. This was mapped onto the CHIME framework in particular, with the suggestion that the arts and creativity can play a role in recovery, with better connections between cultural institutions and recovery-oriented institutions.

## Conclusion

There is a song that I have listened to a lot while working on this project. "Kill the Chord" by the English band Gaffa Tape Sandy (composed of Kim Jarvis, Robin Francis, and Catherine Lindley-Neilson) sums up well the main concepts raised in this chapter (Gaffa Tape Sandy, 2019). The song investigates the creative process, and the judgements laid upon creations:

> Don't let anybody tell you what is and isn't art
> No one can tell you what did and didn't come from the heart

Here, the subjective nature of art and creativity is highlighted. What gives anybody the power to decide what is meaningful? This lyric defends those who are creating, encouraging them not to be dissuaded, and to speak from their heart.

> What's the point in Romanticism?
> Shakespeare, Barocci, and Van Gogh
> What's the point in Georgia O'Keeffe
> Bob Dylan and Michelangelo?

This set of lyrics questions what "the point" of various renowned creatives and artistic movements is. Even the most celebrated works do not have "a point" to Gaffa Tape Sandy. They highlight that these works were made as expression, from a place of emotion and passion. From the soul. There is no need for any greater meaning.

I'm getting sick …
So can we make noise?

Finally, the lyrics take a more personal turn. The band express the value in creativity – how when they are "sick", their instinct is to "make noise", to create. To distract from any problems that they might have, and instead engage in creating music.

Creativity needs not be gatekept, it does not require people to decide whether it is "valuable". Creativity can be a deeply personal expression of the self, and does not require any external meaning greater than that to be considered creative. That is why in times of need, people turn to being creative, to "making noise". It is a human instinct, and as few social boundaries as possible should be put upon that.

It seems clear that, overall, creative therapies have a positive impact on recovery in that they reduce negative affect (Xu et al., 2020). A study by Stickley et al. (2018) combined a literature review with interviews to try and understand how participatory arts were experienced. Their findings were mapped onto the CHIME framework, especially the connectedness and hope dimensions. As well as recovery, inclusion and confidence were felt by participants to have improved.

These studies indicate that creative interventions can help service users with their recovery, which shows that creativity has been applied well to the field of mental health recovery. However, there is seemingly no research into the broader role which creativity plays in the recovery process. For example, in a literature review which in turn examined 67 prior literature reviews on recovery, encompassing a huge amount of data, Ellison et al. (2018) outlined 17 overarching components of recovery. In the text of the article, creativity (and variations of the word) does not appear once.

This, despite all the good that seems to come from creativity in a recovery context. Despite its prevalence in recovery narratives (Hurst et al., 2022). Is creativity the forgotten aspect of recovery? Could it be the confusion between art, talent, and creativity that has led to this oversight? A conceptual confusion between big-C and little-c creativity?

There is a need to understand the experiences of those on a mental health recovery journey and their interactions with creativity.

## References

Amabile, T. M., Barsade, S. G., Mueller, J. S., & Staw, B. M. (2005). Affect and creativity at work. *Administrative Science Quarterly, 50*(*3*), 367–403. doi:10.2189/asqu.2005.50.3.367

Andreasen, N. C. (2006). *The creative brain: The science of genius*. Plume.

Andreasen, N. C., & Ramchandran, K. (2012). Creativity in art and science: Are there two cultures?. *Dialogues in Clinical Neuroscience, 14*(*1*), 49–54. doi:10.31887/DCNS.2012.14.1/nandreasen

Arnout, B. A., & Almoied, A. A. (2021). A structural model relating gratitude, resilience, psychological well-being and creativity among psychological counsellors. *Counselling and Psychotherapy Research, 21*(*2*), 470–488. doi:10.1002/capr.12316

Boardman, J., & Rinaldi, M. (2021). Work, unemployment and mental health. In G. Ikkos & N. Bouras (Eds.), *Mind, state and society: Social history of psychiatry and mental health in Britain 1960–2010* (pp. 326–335). Cambridge University Press.

Burt, E. L., & Atkinson, J. (2012). The relationship between quilting and wellbeing. *Journal of Public Health, 34(1)*, 54–59. doi:10.1093/pubmed/fdr041

Carson, S. H., Peterson, J. B., & Higgins, D. M. (2005). Reliability, validity, and factor structure of the Creative Achievement Questionnaire. *Creativity Research Journal, 17(1)*, 37–50. doi:10.1207/s15326934crj1701_4

Cheung, A., Agwu, V., Stojcevski, M., Wood, L., & Fan, X. (2022). A pilot remote drama therapy program using the co-active therapeutic theater model in people with serious mental illness. *Community Mental Health Journal, 58(8)*, 1613–1620. doi:10.1007/s10597-10022-00977-z

Colbert, S., Cooke, A., Camic, P. M., & Springham, N. (2013). The art-gallery as a resource for recovery for people who have experienced psychosis. *The Arts in Psychotherapy, 40(2)*, 250–256. doi:10.1016/j.aip.2013.03.003.

Csikszentmihalyi, M. (1990). *Flow: The psychology of optimal experience*. Harper & Row.

Damsgaard, J. B., & Jensen, A. (2021). Music activities and mental health recovery: Service users' perspectives presented in the CHIME framework. *International Journal of Environmental Research and Public Health, 18(12)*, 6638. doi:10.3390/ijerph18126638

De Ruysscher, C., Vandevelde, S., Vanheule, S., Bryssinck, D., Haeck, W., & Vanderplasschen, W. (2022). Opening up the black box of recovery processes in persons with complex mental health needs: A qualitative study of place-making dynamics in a low-threshold meeting place. *International Journal of Mental Health Systems, 16(1)*, 50. doi:10.1186/s13033-13022-00560-00569.

Dutton, D. (2006). A naturalist definition of art. *The Journal of Aesthetics and Art Criticism, 64(3)*, 367–377. www.jstor.org/stable/3700568.

Edgell, R. A., & Lee, D. (2023). Theorizing creative challenges: Why are social creativity and reimagined universities necessary for tackling society's problems?. *Journal of Creativity, 33(2)*, 100051. doi:10.1016/j.yjoc.2023.100051

Ellison, M. L., Belanger, L. K., Niles, B. L., Evans, L. C., & Bauer, M. S. (2018). Explication and definition of mental health recovery: A systematic review. *Administration and Policy in Mental Health and Mental Health Services Research, 45(1)*, 91–102. doi:10.1007/s10488-10016-0767-0769.

Fenner, P., Ryan, B., Nabukavou, T., Chang, O., Chetty, S., & Qaloewai, S. (2022). "I function when I'm painting"–Consumers, carers and staff experiences of an art and mental health recovery project in Fiji. *The Arts in Psychotherapy, 77*, 101862. doi:10.1016/j.aip.2021.101862

Fletcher, A., & Benveniste, M. (2022). A new method for training creativity: Narrative as an alternative to divergent thinking. *Annals of the New York Academy of Sciences, 1512(1)*, 29–45. doi:10.1111/nyas.14763

Fletcher, A., Enciso, P., & Benveniste, M. (2023). Narrative creativity training: A new method for increasing resilience in elementary students. *Journal of Creativity, 33(3)*, 100061. doi:10.1016/j.yjoc.2023.100061

Ford, D. Y., & Harris, J. J. (1992). The elusive definition of creativity. *The Journal of Creative Behavior, 26(3)*, 186–198. doi:10.1002/j.2162-6057.1992.tb01175.x

Fritz, B. S., & Avsec, A. (2007). The experience of flow and subjective well-being of music students. *Horizons of Psychology, 16(2)*, 5–17. http://psiholoska-obzorja.si/arhiv_clanki/2007_2/smolej.pdf.

Gaffa Tape Sandy. (2019). Kill the chord [song]. On The Family Mammal. Alcopop! Records.

Gillam, T. (2018). *Creativity, wellbeing and mental health practice*. Springer.

Glăveanu, V. P., & Beghetto, R. A. (2021). Creative experience: A non-standard definition of creativity. *Creativity Research Journal, 33(2)*, 75–80. doi:10.1080/10400419.2020.1827606

Glavin, C. E., & Montgomery, P. (2017). Creative bibliotherapy for post-traumatic stress disorder (PTSD): A systematic review. *Journal of Poetry Therapy, 30(2)*, 95–107. doi:10.1080/08893675.2017.1266190

Goodman-Casanova, J. M., Guzman-Parra, J., Mayoral-Cleries, F., & Cuesta-Lozano, D. (2023). Community-based art groups in mental health recovery: A systematic review and narrative synthesis. *Journal of Psychiatric and Mental Health Nursing, 31(2)*, 158–173. doi:10.1111/jpm.12970

Hansen, B. W., Pedersen, H. A., Brandt, Å., & Berring, L. L. (2023). Creative activities as intervention: experiences of well-being and satisfaction with daily living in a mental health context. *Nordic Journal of Psychiatry, 77(8)*, 788–798. doi:10.1080/08039488.2023.2253236

Hardman, T. J. (2021). Understanding creative intuition. *Journal of Creativity, 31*, 100006. doi:10.1016/j.yjoc.2021.100006

Harrington, D. M. (2018). On the usefulness of "value" in the definition of creativity: A commentary. *Creativity Research Journal, 30(1)*, 118–121. doi:10.1080/10400419.2018.1411432

Henriksen, D., & Shack, K. (2020). Creativity-focused mindfulness for student well-being. *Kappa Delta Pi Record, 56(4)*, 170–175. doi:10.1080/00228958.2020.1813519

Hurst, R., Carson, J., Shahama, A., Kay, H., Nabb, C., & Prescott, J. (2022). Remarkable recoveries: An interpretation of recovery narratives using the CHIME model. *Mental Health and Social Inclusion, 26(2)*, 175–190. doi:10.1108/MHSI-01-2022-0001

Ilha Villanova, A. L., & Pina e Cunha, M. (2021). Everyday creativity: A systematic literature review. *The Journal of Creative Behavior, 55(3)*, 673–695. doi:10.1002/jocb.481

Jay, E. K., Patterson, C., Fernandez, R., & Moxham, L. (2023). Experiences of recovery among adults with a mental illness using visual art methods: A systematic review. *Journal of Psychiatric and Mental Health Nursing, 30(3)*, 361–374. doi:10.1111/jpm.12882

Jensen, A. (2018). Mental health recovery and arts engagement. *The Journal of Mental Health Training, Education and Practice, 13(3)*, 157–166. doi:10.1108/JMHTEP-08-2017-0048

Kaufman, J. C., & Sternberg, R. J. (Eds.). (2010). *The Cambridge handbook of creativity*. Cambridge University Press.

Łucznik, K., May, J., & Redding, E. (2021). A qualitative investigation of flow experience in group creativity. *Research in Dance Education, 22(2)*, 190–209. doi:10.1080/14647893.2020.1746259

Ludowyke, L., Lentin, P., & Brown, T. (2023). The meaning and purpose of creativity in the daily life occupations, activities, acts and behaviors amongst adults living with mental health conditions: A scoping review. *Occupational Therapy in Mental Health, 40(1)*, 45–85. doi:10.1080/0164212X.2023.2218121

Mulatti, C., & Treccani, B. (2023). Perceived lack of control promotes creativity. *Journal of Creativity, 33(1)*, 100040. doi:10.1016/j.yjoc.2022.100040

Mumford, M. D., & England, S. (2022). The future of creativity research: Where are we, and where should we go. *Journal of Creativity, 32(3)*, 100034. doi:10.1016/j.yjoc.2022.100034

Mumford, M. D., & Gustafson, S. B. (1988). Creativity syndrome: Integration, application, and innovation. *Psychological Bulletin, 103*(*1*), 27–43. https://psycnet.apa.org/buy/1988-10128-001.

Nettle, D. (2001). *Strong imagination: Madness, creativity and human nature*. Oxford University Press.

Nitzan, A., & Orkibi, H. (2022). The contribution of integrated arts-based groups to people with mental health conditions and community members: Processes and outcomes. *Psychology of Aesthetics, Creativity, and the Arts*. doi:10.1037/aca0000501

Perkins, R., Ascenso, S., Atkins, L., Fancourt, D., & Williamon, A. (2016). Making music for mental health: How group drumming mediates recovery. *Psychology of Well-being, 6*(*1*), 1–17. doi:10.1186/s13612-13016-0048-0

Peyvastegar, M. (2010). Relationship between creativity and subjective well-being. *International Journal of Behavioral Sciences, 4*(*3*), 207–213. http://www.behavsci.ir/article_67691.html.

Pickering, G. (1974). *Creative malady*. W. & J. Mackay.

Pickover, C. A. (1998). *Strange brains and genius: The secret lives of eccentric scientists and madmen*. Plenum Press.

Pino, M. C., Di Dio, C., Pacitti, F., Rossi, R., Vagnetti, R., Le Donne, I., Marchetti, A., & Mazza, M. (2023). Evaluation of aesthetic pleasure in schizophrenia spectrum disorders, using the eye-tracking methodology. *Psychology of Aesthetics, Creativity, and the Arts, 17*(*1*), 16–28. doi:10.1037/aca0000387

Rankin, J. (2022, September 17). Museums on prescription: Brussels tests cultural visits to treat anxiety. *The Guardian*. https://www.theguardian.com/world/2022/sep/17/museums-on-prescription-brussels-tests-cultural-visits-to-treat-anxiety.

Reid-Wisdom, Z., & Perera-Delcourt, R. (2022). Perceived effects of improv on psychological wellbeing: A qualitative study. *Journal of Creativity in Mental Health, 17*(*2*), 246–263. doi:10.1080/15401383.2020.1856016

Reiter, M. D., Li, P. F., Klee, S., & Sabo, K. (2023). Music in the moment: The use of a musical intervention to impact state experiences. *The Arts in Psychotherapy, 85*, 102053. doi:10.1016/j.aip.2023.102053

Richards, R. (2010). Everyday creativity: Process and way of life – four key issues. In J. C. Kaufman & R. J. Sternberg (Eds.), *The Cambridge handbook of creativity* (pp. 189–215). Cambridge University Press. doi:10.1017/CBO9780511763205.013

Richards, R. (2018). *Everyday creativity and the healthy mind: Dynamic new paths for self and society*. Palgrave Macmillan.

Rogers, C. R. (1967). *On becoming a person*. Constable.

Romm, K. L., Synnes, O., & Bondevik, H. (2022). Creative writing as a means to recover from early psychosis: Experiences from a group intervention. *Arts & Health, 15*(*3*), 292–305. doi:10.1080/17533015.2022.2130379

Rothouse, M. (2023). Navigating the creative wilderness: A depth psychological perspective. *Journal of Creativity, 33*(*2*), 100052. doi:10.1016/j.yjoc.2023.100052

Runco, M. A. (2014). "Big C, little c" creativity as a false dichotomy: Reality is not categorical. *Creativity Research Journal, 26*(*1*), 131–132. doi:10.1080/10400419.2014.873676

Runco, M. A., & Jaeger, G. J. (2012). The standard definition of creativity. *Creativity Research Journal, 24*(*1*), 92–96. doi:10.1080/10400419.2012.650092

Ryan, B., Fenner, P., Chang, O., Qaloewai, S., Nabukavou, T., & Chetty, S. (2021). Art-making in mental health–a Fijian pilot study. *Australasian Psychiatry, 29*(*2*), 204–206. doi:10.1177/1039856220970060

Salomon-Gimmon, M. (2023). "A springboard back to life": The voices of people with mental health conditions on the process and outcomes of a pre-academic arts program. *The Arts in Psychotherapy, 85*, 102054. doi:10.1016/j.aip.2023.102054

Sawyer, R. K. (2011). *Explaining creativity: The science of human innovation.* Oxford University Press.

Sawyer, R. K. (2021). The iterative and improvisational nature of the creative process. *Journal of Creativity, 31*, 100002. doi:10.1016/j.yjoc.2021.100002

Schutte, N. S., & Malouff, J. M. (2020). Connections between curiosity, flow and creativity. *Personality and Individual Differences, 152*, 109555. doi:10.1016/j.paid.2019.109555

Shaw, A. (2023). Creative Minecrafters: Cognitive and personality determinants of creativity, novelty, and usefulness in Minecraft. *Psychology of Aesthetics, Creativity, and the Arts, 17(1)*, 106–117. doi:10.1037/aca0000456

Silverman, M. J. (2019). Comparing educational music therapy interventions via stages of recovery with adults in an acute care mental health setting: A cluster-randomized pilot effectiveness study. *Community Mental Health Journal, 55(4)*, 624–630. doi:10.1007/s10597-10019-00380-00381.

Slanzi, C. M., Brusilovskiy, E., McCormick, B., Snethen, G., & Salzer, M. S. (2023). Participation in arts and culture among individuals with serious mental illnesses and its relationship to quality of life and recovery. *Psychiatric Rehabilitation Journal, 46(2)*, 117. doi:10.1037/prj0000553

Smedley, D., & Croffie, A. L. (2023). The power of vulnerability: Connecting families using Spider-man: Into the Spider-Verse. *Journal of Creativity in Mental Health, 18(2)*, 277–287. doi:10.1080/15401383.2021.1960667

Stewart, V., Roennfeldt, H., Slattery, M., & Wheeler, A. J. (2019). Generating mutual recovery in creative spaces. *Mental Health and Social Inclusion, 23(1)*, 16–22. doi:10.1108/MHSI-08-2018-0029

Stickley, T., Wright, N., & Slade, M. (2018). The art of recovery: Outcomes from participatory arts activities for people using mental health services. *Journal of Mental Health, 27(4)*, 367–373. doi:10.1080/09638237.2018.1437609

Storr, A. (1993). *The dynamics of creation.* Penguin Books.

Sui, T. Y., McDermott, S., Harris, B., & Hsin, H. (2023). The impact of physical environments on outpatient mental health recovery: A design-oriented qualitative study of patient perspectives. *PLoS ONE, 18(4)*, e0283962. doi:10.1371/journal.pone.0283962

Tan, C. Y., Chuah, C. Q., Lee, S. T., & Tan, C. S. (2021). Being creative makes you happier: The positive effect of creativity on subjective well-being. *International Journal of Environmental Research and Public Health, 18(14)*, 7244. doi:10.3390/ijerph18147244

Treffert, D. A. (1989). *Extraordinary people: An exploration of the Savant syndrome.* Transworld Publishers.

Tribe, K. V., Papps, F. A., & Calvert, F. (2021). "It just gives people hope": A qualitative inquiry into the lived experience of the Harry Potter world in mental health recovery. *The Arts in Psychotherapy, 74*, 101802. doi:10.1016/j.aip.2021.101802

Van Lith, T. (2014). "Painting to find my spirit": Art making as the vehicle to find meaning and connection in the mental health recovery process. *Journal of Spirituality in Mental Health, 16(1)*, 19–36. doi:10.1080/19349637.2013.864542

Vyas, M. (2021). Experience of flow in games and using it to improve well-being: A critical review. *Indian Journal of Health & Wellbeing, 12(1)*. https://iahrw.org/our-services/journals/indian-journal-of-health-wellbeing/.

Vygotsky, L. S. (2004). Imagination and creativity in childhood. *Journal of Russian & East European Psychology, 42*, 7–97. doi:10.1080/10610405.2004.11059210

Walia, C. (2019). A dynamic definition of creativity. *Creativity Research Journal, 31(3)*, 237–247. doi:10.1080/10400419.2019.1641787

Wang, S., Bressington, D. T., Leung, A. Y. M., Davidson, P. M., & Cheung, D. S. K. (2020). The effects of bibliotherapy on the mental well-being of informal caregivers of people with neurocognitive disorder: A systematic review and meta-analysis. *International Journal of Nursing Studies, 109*, 103643. doi:10.1016/j.ijnurstu.2020.103643

Ward, S. J., & King, L. A. (2017). Work and the good life: How work contributes to meaning in life. *Research in Organizational Behavior, 37*, 59–82. doi:10.1016/j.riob.2017.10.001

Weisberg, R. W. (2006). *Creativity: Understanding innovation in problem solving, science, invention, and the arts.* John Wiley & Sons.

Weisberg, R. W. (2015). On the usefulness of "value" in the definition of creativity. *Creativity Research Journal, 27(2)*, 111–124. doi:10.1080/10400419.2015.1030320

Williams, E., Dingle, G. A., Calligeros, R., Sharman, L., & Jetten, J. (2020). Enhancing mental health recovery by joining arts-based groups: A role for the social cure approach. *Arts & Health, 12(2)*, 169–181. doi:10.1080/17533015.2019.1624584

Xu, L., Cheng, P., Wu, Y., Zhang, J., Zhu, J., Cui, J., & Yu, R. (2020). The effects of art therapy on anxiety and depression in breast cancer patients: An updated meta-analysis. *European Journal of Cancer Care, 29(5)*, e13266. doi:10.1111/ecc.13266

Zhang, D. D., Bennett, M. R., Cheng, H., Wang, L., Zhang, H., Reynolds, S. C., Zhang, S., Wang, X., Li, T., Urban, T., Pei, Q., Wu, Z., Zhang, P., Liu, C., Wang, Y., Wang, C., Zhang, D., & Edwards, R. L. (2021). Earliest parietal art: Hominin hand and foot traces from the middle Pleistocene of Tibet. *Science Bulletin, 66(24)*, 2506–2515. doi:10.1016/j.scib.2021.09.001

# 5 What has brought us here?

*Robert Hurst, Andrew Voyce, and Jerome Carson*

So far, we have justified our investigations into creativity and recovery using academic sources. These have of course influenced us in our approaches to studying these topics. However, what personal reasons brought us here?

By giving you this context, we hope you will be able to see why we interpreted things in the ways that we did, and transfer some epistemic power back to readers who can then decide for themselves the quality of our analyses (Gyollai, 2020).

Autoethnography is a methodology that allows researchers to bring their Self into the research (Poulos, 2021). It asks a question – why does my story only have validity if I am asked about it by somebody else (Wall, 2008)? Using autoethnography, we describe our Selves within our respective settings (Poerwandari, 2021). We each bring a unique viewpoint. Andrew as an ex-asylum-patient, Jerome as a retired clinical psychologist and current Professor of Psychology, and Robert as an early career psychology academic with a history of using creativity for healing.

In this chapter, we endeavour to show readers why we, as researchers, are studying creativity in mental health recovery. We will then outline how we conducted our study.

## Our stories

### Jerome Carson

Truth be told, I have never really considered myself to be a creative person. I suppose I associated creativity with artistic creativity and, having been awarded a poor grade in O level art, it was a gift I felt I never possessed. Working with Robert has of course taught me that creativity is much broader than this.

In 2006, I was given a "free transfer" from the Institute of Psychiatry to the South London and Maudsley NHS Trust. Having to leave was one of the lowest points of my career. In a meeting with my mentor, I was assured I could keep my title. I immediately countered that I would not, as it would only be an "honorary title". Despite being a massive blow to my self-esteem, it made me determined to make a real difference with what I did next in my career. I suppose I was full of the

DOI: 10.4324/9781003319405-5

"righteous indignation" described by Pat Deegan. At the time I had no idea that the area I would make my mark in was mental health recovery.

So, in September 2006, I arrived to work as the consultant clinical psychologist at a community mental health team base. It had just been divided into two functional teams – "Assessment and Treatment", and "Recovery and Support". As the only consultant clinical psychologist at the team base, I was to work across both teams. Both had been assembled almost overnight. One day they had one set of functions, the next they had new functions. My inclination was to focus more on recovery and support. I could see that I had the possibility of shaping the philosophy of this new team. One of the first things I set up was a series of education sessions. While these were helpful, the real transformation came when I started working in partnership with people who used our services (Carson, 2012).

It is strange how things can happen serendipitously in life. One of the things I had done for my PhD was to run workshops on self-esteem for staff. I decided to run some for people who used our services. I was due to put on an event for World Mental Health Day, and one of the workshop participants asked if she could display her artwork. Her work was inspiring and showed how creative she was. I asked her to do a presentation at the team base to both people who used our service as well as staff and students. This was the start of our Recovery Group (Morgan & Carson, 2009). The next presentation was by the film-maker Michelle McNary, who gave a presentation entitled "Recovery from mental illness: Do service users hold the keys to our understanding?". The third involved me interviewing Gordon McManus in front of an audience about his own model of recovery (McManus, 2012). Dolly Sen was the inspirational fourth presenter (Sen, 2002).

These workshops offered our local service users the chance to talk about an area they had excelled in, often art- or craft-related. In a sense, I was capturing the creativity of local people. We also invited several lived experience experts from around the UK to come and inspire local people, including Dr Peter Chadwick, Peter Bullimore, Dr Rachel Perkins, and our own Andrew Voyce. Peter Chadwick attracted an audience of 50 people, who packed into the group room of the team base as he gave an electrifying performance on his views of psychosis (Chadwick, 2011). Over five years, I worked with people with lived experience and a number of assistant psychologists and multidisciplinary colleagues to deliver a whole series of initiatives around creativity and recovery. These included:

- Making a film about recovery, led by Michelle McNary (Carson et al., 2012; Maudsley NHS, 2010).
- Helping Matt Ward (an actor) put on a series of plays.
- Three World Mental Health Day events on the theme of mental health recovery.
- A one-day conference at the Institute of Psychiatry, with a book launch.
- Helping many individuals get charitable grants to enable them to work on their own recovery.
- The publication of the Recovery Heroes series (Sen et al., 2009; Chadwick et al., 2009; McManus et al., 2009; Ward et al., 2010; Muir et al., 2010).

- A series of four papers on Historical Recovery Heroes, co-authored with Liz Wakely (Wakely & Carson 2010; Wakely & Carson, 2011a; Wakely & Carson, 2011b; Wakely & Carson, 2011c).
- Three books on mental health recovery, all co-authored with people with lived experience, (Cordle et al., 2011; Davies et al., 2011; McManus & Carson, 2012).

My creativity was in coming up with all of these diverse ideas, but to a large extent all of these activities tapped into the creativity of the people with lived experience of mental illness and their subsequent recovery, which the activities above illustrated. I am not sure if Andrew will remember his visit to our recovery group. He was so brimming with ideas and excitement himself, that he actually gave us three talks and not one!

This was probably the most creative period of my clinical career. However, the model was not sustainable. I took on too much of this work myself, with largely only the help of assistant psychologists. Before Matt Ward's set of plays, I had all my family help put together the educational handouts that we provided for the audiences. At the same time, I was still having to do all my clinical work. This exhaustion, combined with some setbacks, led to my decision to retire from the NHS in 2011. My retirement party was held in the Atrium at Guy's Hospital and was attended by over 100 people. More than a third of attendees were people with lived experience. It was a memorable event, perhaps let down by a 30-minute speech from me? I had a lot of people to thank. Indeed, I did.

*Andrew Voyce*

Do I hear voices? No I don't, despite my surname.

But have I had strange non-consensual thoughts and views of reality? Yes, most definitely.

These false beliefs, delusions, are described under the heading of schizophrenia. I concur with that. I am also happy that a therapeutic dose of atypical antipsychotic medication has coincided with 30 years without arrest or inpatient episode, and with no feelings of paranoia, and no strange beliefs that no-one else shares. However, I do not agree with the medical view of schizophrenia. Thomas Szasz (1961), Michel Foucault (2001) and others make extremely cogent arguments that mental illness should not be a descriptor. Schizophrenia and other conditions are not illnesses and should not be described or treated as such.

The paradox is that a daily pill has coincided with a good life for me, symptom free. Yet I find the treatment of psychiatric disorders by medical experts somewhat absurd. There is a whole medically based paraphernalia from diagnosis all the way to the labels on boxes in the nurse's room, and yet quite often this process does not have a beneficial effect on the patient. Why does care take place thus, I ask. Surely there is a better way. Why should it be that 10mg daily of Olanzapine atypical antipsychotic should be so beneficial for me, even though there is no complete paradigm to explain why this should be so.

Therefore, am I saying that the medical model of psychiatry should be replaced by a model of creativity? Most definitely not. For me, current versions of recovery models offer practical insight into improvements from mental health issues, and mirror my experiences. Where a symptom-free life can be brought about, or where symptoms can be coped with, there is a possibility of moving beyond the life of a mental patient and finding a place in society. For me it is helpful to replace the medical hegemony with a focus on recovery; and with a recovery-oriented pathway, creativity becomes for some a way of getting a sense of self.

That has certainly been true for me. I have not been content to sit around and revel in 30 years without arrest or time on an inpatient ward. That is not for me. I have found an outlet in creativity that has helped me to make sense of 20 lost years as a psychiatric revolving door patient. Partly or wholly, a creative life of statement has led me through dependency on welfare benefits to a life of independence. For me this in itself is another manifestation of a creative process. As well as an interest in what most people will describe as creativity, I have an academic background in social science. I have experienced that also as a creative endeavour. I have attempted to live up to societal norms, and I have challenged circumstances to make this so. This has had creative aspects.

It pleased me immensely to grow sunflowers in a social services garden. From that I derived my logo, which is a mock-up of Van Gogh's vase of sunflowers using real sunflowers I grew and a papier-mâché container, alongside Vincent's painting; all in a side-by-side photograph. Creatively copying sunflowers. If my life is not in some part about C-CHIME, what is it about?

I think it is clear that writing about recovery aspects of my life, and recognising affinity in the lives and statements of others, comes intuitively to me. Some things are self-evident to all of us, and other things are not part of our ready vocabulary. For me, recovery is a friendly and helpful part of mental health services, I have to say that I do not find all of service delivery to be so. Mental health is a contested field (McCabe et al., 2018), where the institutional establishment is so very hard to get on-side with progressive practice. Principles such as treatment needing to be therapeutic (enshrined in the 2017 Review of the Mental Health Act; UK Government, 2018), person-centred approaches, and positive risk-taking are not always evident in twenty-first-century mental health services. In fact, quite the opposite. So, recovery-focused practice appeals to me and drew me into this project. In particular, creativity has given me my voice (as is my surname) in a community that I feel a belonging to. I have to say that a completely dulled life as a revolving door patient is something, looking back, that I find hard to explain. How did I get there? My creativity helped me begin to start answering that question.

When I was invited to co-author this project, I felt honoured and humbled. Maybe they are not the entirety of my life, but the recovery movement and creativity have been important to me for a number of years. How I got to be embedded in the asylum system is indeed a travesty, but today I am happy that there are many good people in the mental health system. I feel an empathy with my co-authors.

What I can say is that you can end up in a happy place. In fact, the longer I lead a life of independence and responsibility, the more secure I feel that it will continue.

To summarise, I have to say I would have liked to have produced art that is valued for stand-alone merit. Rather, my creative output has been to tell an untold story which has enabled me to move on from difficult episodes. As Maya Angelou is quoted as saying – "There is no greater agony than bearing an untold story inside you" (as referenced by Kim, 2017). Creativity has allowed me to lighten the load, and share my story in my words.

### Robert Hurst

In my life, I have been lucky enough to travel to some amazing places, to see amazing things. Recently, with my head in this project, I have been looking out for creativity, for the huge effect that it can have. One place that I have visited is the Uffizi Museum in Florence, Italy. This is an art gallery hosting works of Renaissance geniuses. Da Vinci, Botticelli, Michelangelo, Gentileschi, and countless others. The aesthetic beauty of these works was indescribable. Vibrant colours, perfectly carved marble. To see those masterpieces with my own eyes was something entirely unique. It felt almost spiritual, and affected me in profound, emotional ways. Experiencing those works of creativity made me feel amazing. It had an impact on me.

Two years later, I was in Tallinn, Estonia. This is a nation that is less than 40 years removed from being a Soviet state, and the horrors that came along with that. While there, I visited a former prison which housed Estonian dissenters of the regime. This moved me in an entirely different way. While the walls were crumbling, posters and etchings still remained in the cells. The place felt lived in... haunted. One of the exhibits elevated this sense of walking among ghosts.

There was a room, which once housed prisoners, filled with dim bulbs. On the lampshades were images of objects, with a paragraph describing them. Each was something that had been made by the prisoners while incarcerated. There were illicit Christmas cards, love poems, knitted Estonian flags. These were much less technically and aesthetically appealing than the masterpieces in the Uffizi. And yet as I dodged the bedframes on which the prisoners once slept, examining each object, I was more emotionally moved. I found the creations just as breathtakingly beautiful because of the stories behind them.

The purpose of our creativity can be to achieve beauty. It can also be to survive. To have an outlet. To leave something of ourselves behind in the physical world. A small act of rebellion in absurd circumstances.

My experiences with creativity have been profound. In times of difficulty, I have always found myself turning in some way to creativity. Sometimes that is by being creative myself, other times it was by consuming works of creativity.

My own creative force has also been a vital part of my emotional first aid kit. Throughout my life, I have had various creative interests that have fuelled my sense of meaning and brought me joy – from writing stories as a child, to creating website projects as a young adult. These are things that I have loved doing. However, sometimes, these creative endeavours have saved me.

This is particularly true of music. I learned to play the guitar as a teenager, and this has at many points been a life jacket for me. It is now the most important tool in my arsenal when it comes to getting a grasp on my emotions when in crisis. A particularly strong example comes from when I went through a dark time personally. I was lucky enough to have wonderful friends who would listen to me talk about how I felt for hours on end. While this was cathartic, there also was an itch that could only be scratched through my creativity. And so I wrote, I crafted, I sung, I played, I laboured. I let the music flow through me, and put pieces of my soul into it along the way.

Writing songs was a precious outlet, a means of expression like no other available to me. Through the lyrics I could say things in a way that felt meaningful, the rhythm and tone of the words adding something more to the underlying meanings of them. Then there was the crafting of melodies and chord progressions. There was something in the notes behind the lyrics that could capture those emotions which were beyond my vocabulary. Those ineffable feelings that can't be put into words, I was able to bring to life through my songs. This was creativity as therapy, for me. The catharsis was intense. I have shared very few of my songs with anybody – this was not a way of capitalising on my sadness for any artistic merit. It was a channelling of emotion. It worked for me.

However, as mentioned earlier, I think that consuming the creations of others can also have a big impact. Sticking with music, listening to songs has always been something of a mood regulator for me personally. It can help me to wallow in low moods, raise me up when I need a boost, relax me when things are too much, and help me feel utterly ecstatic. There really is a song for each mood.

I was reminded of this while writing this chapter. Taking a walk, I was listening to a band that I hadn't heard for some years. Each song unlocked a fresh set of emotional memories for me. I could remember being in the car-ride home after seeing the band for the first time. I could picture listening to songs in specific places, sharing them with specific people. I remember going to see them perform with a close friend, hearing particular songs played live. This was all relatively pedestrian, very enjoyable. The usual level of sentimentality that I experience fairly often.

Until one particular song began to play.

As the verse entered the chorus, I could *feel* the song. Chills ran down my back, tendrils of locked-away emotion scuttled across my arms. Instinctively mouthing along, tears formed in my eyes. I had listened to this song a lot at a particular time in my life, a difficult and lonely one. While the song reminded me of that time, it did not cause me pain. The tears were not of sadness, but of… . Well, I am not so sure. Perhaps melancholy? Whatever it was, it was not an unpleasant thing to feel. It brought out a strong emotion, which felt cathartic. I could almost feel dopamine surge through my ventricles. It was a physical as well as an emotive experience.

Does that tie into recovery? That is not a question that I feel comfortable answering alone. However, the experience reminded me why consuming the creativity of others is an important aspect of wellbeing. When that band wrote and then produced this song, this audible artifact, they were infusing it with their own emotions and meanings. Their own experiences. By the time it got to me, much of that was lost. But it didn't matter. Whatever original intent was left in the lyrics and the melodic, rhythmic *feel* of the song, I picked up on what mattered to me and brought my own meaning to it.

I wrote this to share an in-depth experience. I chose it due to recency, as I could give a rich account. But music has undoubtedly had this effect upon me often. Many times, it has saved me. Pulled me through otherwise impossible moments of anguish and pain. A life raft in turbulent seas of emotion. In tough times, songs filled with anger and heartbreak made me feel heard and understood. Happy, uplifting songs at that time did not interest me. Eventually though, they did, and I was able to move to a better place, with a helping hand from the music.

That is my interest in this project. I have always had this underlying curiosity in the power of creativity. When analysing the data in our second review of Remarkable Lives papers (Hurst et al., 2022), this predisposed sense of creativity as a force for healing may have unconsciously made me more perceptive of the way that creativity was present in the accounts. I may have noticed it in those participants because I have felt it in myself. Though this research was conducted with a team, giving the data more reliability, as I was not alone in making that interpretation. However, I was conscious of these biases as I embarked on the work for this project. I did my best to focus on what the StoryTellers brought, on what creativity has meant to them in their mental health recovery. I wanted to be challenged and be shown a different side of creativity. I was not disappointed.

I adore John Berger's *Ways of Seeing*. He takes the often-elitist topic of art, and he tries to make it appeal to everyone. He does not speak down, nor does he try to obfuscate or gatekeep. In many ways, in its style it was the blueprint for this project for me. With this book I am attempting to do for creativity what John Berger attempted to do for art all those years ago. I want to try and show people that creativity is for everyone. It is for me, it is for you, it is for every single person that you know. Each of us will have our own unique approach and that is fine. In fact, it is wonderful!

What drew me to this project was a lifetime of experience, of noticing just how much my creativity and the creative works of others have helped me with my mental health. As I began to read, I became further motivated by a desire to compassionately disrupt the current ideas about creativity. I want to make my contribution to emancipating creativity from cultural gatekeepers. Perhaps somewhat ambitious, but that was my driving force, alongside helping people to understand how creativity can help, how it can hinder, and encouraging readers to reflect on their own creativity and the impacts that it has on their lives.

## Methods

Having now presented readers with our philosophical, theoretical, and personal backgrounds for this work, the stage is set for our StoryTellers. Just before we get to them, let us introduce the methods we used.

*Study design*

To attempt to understand how creativity is experienced within the context of mental health recovery, interpretative phenomenological analysis (IPA) was chosen as the methodology for this study. IPA is based on Husserl's idea of phenomenology (Smith & Nizza, 2022), that to understand what underlies a concept, you must strip away your ideas as much as possible to "go back to the things themselves" (Husserl, 2001, p. 168). To understand the essence of something, we must try to put our existing knowledge to one side – "bracket" it (Dowling & Cooney, 2012). In other words, IPA attempts to approach topics with an open mind.

Data collection was approached with an awareness of trying to understand experiences in a bottom-up way (Reid et al., 2005). We felt that doing this returned some power to the participants. This is reflected in the semi-structured interview format that was used (Smith, 2017). Robert would go into each interview with a loose set of questions, intended to spark discussion and allow for each interviewee to lead the conversation as much as possible.

Another way to bracket our experiences is by understanding this approach as double hermeneutic. The epistemological stance of IPA is a hermeneutic one (Smith et al., 2009) – understanding is arrived at by making an interpretation (Heidegger, 1962). In IPA's case, the interpretation is "local", made by the researcher (Smith & Nizza, 2022). Therefore, to acknowledge that fundamental meaning-making role of the researcher makes the output of IPA double hermeneutic – it is the researcher's interpretation of the participant's interpretations of their experiences (Giddens, 1987). This makes us active participants in the research; from the formulation of the research question to the interviews to the interpretation; we brought our own experiences and biases (Biggerstaff & Thompson, 2008).

As completely avoiding bringing in prior personal experience when interpreting data is impossible in practice (Gyollai, 2020), the only way to bracket it is to acknowledge it (Sydor, 2019). That is what this chapter has aimed to achieve. Context is important, as IPA is not simply a method of analysis, but informs each stage of the research process – including the afterlife of the analysis. You, as the reader, will conduct your own analysis. You may agree with our interpretations, or make your own.

Some readers may wonder what validity this methodology had – did it accurately measure what it is to use creativity within mental health recovery? On this point, it is important to consider that IPA is an idiographic approach. Rather than seeking to achieve empirical generalisability (Wagstaff et al., 2014), it is concerned with what it is to be human, with the particular (Vicary et al., 2017). Similarly with reliability, the methodology is concerned with participants' interpretations (and the researchers' interpretation of these) rather than with empirical "truth". The reliability of participant narratives are taken as a given, and we have endeavoured to interpret the data in good faith. In this way, the results presented are a reliable account of the interview and analysis process.

IPA has previously been used to study creativity in the context of mental health, but the focus was not specifically on the experience of creativity within mental health recovery. Rather, other studies have examined participant experiences of various creative therapies such as art therapy (Fenner et al., 2022) and music therapy (Perkins et al., 2016). This does not tell us what the role of creativity is in individual mental health recovery in a broad context. Therefore, the present work sought to fill this gap in knowledge, using IPA to explore broadly the experiences that five individuals had of creativity within mental health recovery.

### Participants

The study involved five "participants" – our StoryTellers. We used opportunity sampling when choosing our five. This is a method for gathering participants where you ask specific people to be involved, because you know that they have the relevant insight and experiences to be able to contribute rich, relevant data to the study (Smith & Osborn, 2003). It would be no use randomly selecting people to get involved. We needed those involved in the study to a) be able to talk on the topic of mental health recovery, having had experiences with the concept themselves, and b) for them to be creative individuals in some way. With these being the two areas interrogated by the study, it was imperative to get people involved who would be a good fit. The small sample size is usual for an IPA study, as the goal is in-depth analysis of individuals' experiences (Pietkiewicz & Smith, 2014).

### Collection of data

Interviews with the StoryTellers were conducted over Zoom by Robert. He served as the interviewer and conducted the IPA analysis. As mentioned, interview questions were kept open-ended, allowing room for participants to explore their experiences in-depth with little directing from the researcher (Smith, 2011).

The interviews lasted between 50 and 90 minutes. Once completed, the researcher created a typed transcript of each interview manually, so as to get a deeper understanding of and connection with the data. These were sent to the StoryTellers, giving them an opportunity to elaborate on or correct anything. Interviews began in February 2022 and were spaced at least one week apart to allow time for reflection on each interview, and any necessary adjustments to be made to questions.

### Analysis of data

Each transcript was first analysed individually. The analysis was done in a line-by-line way to ensure that no data was missed (Smith & Nizza, 2022). From each interview, a rough set of categories was formed. From the second interview onwards, as well as an individual analysis, previous cases were incorporated to create an evolving cross-case analysis. Afterwards, the resulting model was checked against each individual StoryTeller to ensure as much consistency as possible. Alongside this process, Robert was maintaining an awareness of his own interpretations and attempting to log and then bracket these from the initial analysis.

Once a rough set of categories was arrived at, Robert incorporated some of his own interpretations into the model – embracing the double hermeneutic nature of IPA and interpreting the interpretations made by the participants. This allowed for a cohesive narrative and model to be created, to best fit all of the five StoryTellers' experiences.

The study was written up in the scientific format. Analyses were made, and a model was created to visualise how we interpreted creativity in recovery. That is a description of the study we conducted, but creating the stories for this book included extra steps.

### *Preparation of StoryTeller chapters*

We did not want to leave readers with five interview transcripts to read through. That format does not do the stories justice. The approach we decided to take was for Robert to take each transcript and weave it into a story. Taking all of the key elements and insights of the StoryTellers and putting them into one, cohesive, readable piece. This approach is borrowed from Julie Leibrich's book *A Gift of Stories* (Leibrich, 1999). Julie interviewed various service users from around New Zealand about their lived experience. She then wrote up their stories using her StoryTellers' own words. When a draft was ready, she would send it to be checked and changed as the StoryTeller saw fit. This is what we have attempted to do. Robert is writing up the story to ensure some stylistic cohesion, the StoryTellers are checking it to make sure it represents their experiences.

Throughout this process, we have taken great care to avoid "narrative entrapment" (Grant, 2018) – trapping somebody into a story that they have no power over. We have no desire to colonise the stories of our StoryTellers. They have chosen to share them. We are deeply grateful for that. We believe that sharing these stories will be beneficial to readers. This is why we have asked for their input on their chapters, and on the overall picture of what we are presenting. They have been kind and supportive throughout.

### *Structure of StoryTeller chapters*

The StoryTeller chapters will all follow a similar format. Firstly, we will introduce the StoryTeller with a little background on how we came to initially meet them, and why we asked them to be involved. Then, the stories. Finally, Robert will briefly comment on what each StoryTeller added to his thinking, how they shaped the research. The final overall analysis will be presented in Chapter 12, bringing the input of the five StoryTellers together to form a cohesive model for the ways that creativity can operate in recovery.

So, are you sitting comfortably? Good. Then we will begin.

### References

Biggerstaff, D., & Thompson, A. R. (2008). Interpretative phenomenological analysis (IPA): A qualitative methodology of choice in healthcare research. *Qualitative Research in Psychology*, 5(3), 214–224. doi:10.1080/14780880802314304.

Carson, J. (2012). Recovery from mental illness: A personal journey and a look at recovery from top to bottom. In G. McManus & J. Carson (Eds.), *From communism to schizophrenia and beyond: One man's long march to recovery* (pp. 99–128). Whiting and Birch.

Carson, J., McNary, M., Wolfson, P., & Holloway, F. (2012). The making of a film about recovery. *Mental Health and Social Inclusion, 16*(2), 72–78. doi:10.1108/20428301211232478.

Chadwick, P. (2011). *Schizophrenia the positive perspective: Explorations at the outer reaches of human experience*. Routledge.

Chadwick, P., Morgan, S., Fradgley, J., & Carson, J. (2009). Recovery heroes: A profile of Peter Chadwick. *A Life in the Day, 13*(3), 6–9. doi:10.1108/13666282200900024.

Cordle, H., Fradgley, J., Carson, J., Holloway, F., & Richards, P. (Eds.) (2011). *Psychosis: Stories of recovery and hope*. Quay Books.

Davies, S., Wakely, E., Morgan, S., & Carson, J. (Eds.) (2011). *Mental health recovery heroes past and present*. Pavilion Publishing.

Dowling, M., & Cooney, A. (2012). Research approaches related to phenomenology: Negotiating a complex landscape. *Nurse Researcher, 20*(2). doi:10.7748/nr2012.11.20.2.21.c9440.

Fenner, P., Ryan, B., Nabukavou, T., Chang, O., Chetty, S., & Qaloewai, S. (2022). "I function when I'm painting"– Consumers, carers and staff experiences of an art and mental health recovery project in Fiji. *The Arts in Psychotherapy, 77*, 101862. doi:10.1016/j.aip.2021.101862.

Foucault, M. (2001). *Madness and civilisation*. Routledge.

Giddens, A. (1987). *Social theory and modern sociology*. Stanford University Press.

Grant, A. (2018). Introduction: Voice, ethics, and the best of autoethnographic intentions (Or writers, readers, and the spaces in-between). In L. Turner, N. P. Short, A. Grant & T. E. Adams (Eds.), *International perspectives on autoethnographic research and practice* (pp. 105–122). Routledge.

Gyollai, D. (2020). Getting into it in the wrong way: Interpretative phenomenological analysis and the hermeneutic circle. *Nursing Philosophy, 21*(2), e12294. doi:10.1111/nup.12294.

Heidegger, M. (1962). *Being and time* (J. Macquarrie & E. Robinson, Trans.). SCM Press. (Original work published 1927.)

Hurst, R., Carson, J., Shahama, A., Kay, H., Nabb, C., & Prescott, J. (2022). Remarkable recoveries: An interpretation of recovery narratives using the CHIME model. *Mental Health and Social Inclusion, 26*(2), 175–190. doi:10.1108/MHSI-01-2022-0001.

Husserl, E. (2001). *Logical investigations*, volume *I* (J. Findlay, trans.). Routledge. (Original work published 1900.)

Kim, J. H. (2017). Autobiography as Foucauldian askēsis: Care of the self and care of others. *a/b: Auto/Biography Studies, 32*(2), 327–329. doi:10.1080/08989575.2017.1288968.

Leibrich, J. (1999). *A gift of stories: Discovering how to deal with mental illness*. University of Otago Press.

Maudsley NHS. (2010). Recovery and mental illness: Part one [video]. www.youtube.com/watch?v=purscrXmygc.

McCabe, R., Whittington, R., Cramond, L., & Perkins, E. (2018). Contested understandings of recovery in mental health. *Journal of Mental Health, 27*(5), 475–481. doi:10.1080/09638237.2018.1466037.

McManus, G. (2012). My journey of recovery. In G. McManus & J. Carson (Eds.), *From communism to schizophrenia and beyond: One man's long march to recovery* (pp. 41–54). Whiting and Birch.

McManus, G., & Carson, J. (Eds.) (2012). *From communism to schizophrenia and beyond: One man's long march to recovery*. Whiting and Birch.

McManus, G., Morgan, S., Fradgley, J., & Carson, J. (2009). Recovery heroes: A profile of Gordon McManus. *A Life in the Day*, *13*(*4*), 16–19. doi:10.1108/13666282200900037.

Morgan, S., & Carson, J. (2009). The recovery group: A service user and professional perspective. *Groupwork*, *19*(*1*), 26–39. https://journals.whitingbirch.net/index.php/GPWK/article/view/662.

Muir, M., Cordle, H., & Carson, J. (2010). Recovery heroes: A profile of Margaret Muir. *Mental Health and Social Inclusion*, *14*(*2*), 7–11. doi:10.5042/mhsi.2010.0235.

Perkins, R., Ascenso, S., Atkins, L., Fancourt, D., & Williamon, A. (2016). Making music for mental health: How group drumming mediates recovery. *Psychology of Well-being*, *6*(*1*), 1–17. doi:10.1186/s13612-016-0048-0.

Pietkiewicz, I., & Smith, J. A. (2014). A practical guide to using interpretative phenomenological analysis in qualitative research psychology. *Psychological Journal*, *20*(*1*), 7–14. doi:10.14691/CPPJ.20.1.7.

Poerwandari, E. K. (2021). Minimizing bias and maximizing the potential strengths of autoethnography as a narrative research. *Japanese Psychological Research*, *63*(*4*), 310–323. doi:10.1111/jpr.12320.

Poulos, C. N. (2021). Conceptual foundations of autoethnography. In C. N. Poulos (Ed.), *Essentials of autoethnography* (pp. 3–17). American Psychological Association. doi:10.1037/0000222-001.

Reid, K., Flowers, P., & Larkin, M. (2005). Exploring lived experience. *The Psychologist*, *18*(*1*), 20–23. https://psycnet.apa.org/record/2005-02203-005.

Sen, D. (2002). *The world is full of laughter*. Chipmunka Publishing.

Sen, D., Morgan, S., & Carson, J. (2009). Recovery heroes: A profile of Dolly Sen. *A Life in the Day*, *13*(*2*), 6–8. doi:10.1108/13666282200900013.

Smith, J. A. (2011). Evaluating the contribution of interpretative phenomenological analysis. *Health Psychology Review*, *5*(*1*), 9–27. doi:10.1080/17437199.2010.510659.

Smith, J. A. (2017). Interpretative phenomenological analysis: Getting at lived experience. *The Journal of Positive Psychology*, *12*(*3*), 303–304. doi:10.1080/17439760.2016.1262622.

Smith, J. A., & Nizza, I. E. (2022). *Essentials of Interpretative Phenomenological Analysis*. American Psychological Association.

Smith, J. A. & Osborn, M. (2003). Interpretative phenomenological analysis. In J. A. Smith (Ed.), *Qualitative Psychology: A practical guide to research methods* (pp. 51–80). Sage.

Smith, J. A., Flowers, P., & Larkin, M. (2009). *Interpretative phenomenological analysis: Theory, method and research*. Sage Publications.

Sydor, A. (2019). An interpretative phenomenological analysis of young men's experiences of addressing their sexual health and the importance of researcher reflexivity. *Journal of Research in Nursing*, *24*(*1–2*), 36–46. doi:10.1177/1744987118818865.

Szasz, T. (1961). *The myth of mental illness*. Secker & Warburg.

UK Government. (2018). Independent Review of the Mental Health Act. www.gov.uk/government/groups/independent-review-of-the-mental-health-act.

Vicary, S., Young, A., & Hicks, S. (2017). A reflective journal as learning process and contribution to quality and validity in interpretative phenomenological analysis. *Qualitative Social Work*, *16*(*4*), 550–565. doi:10.1177/1473325016635244.

Wagstaff, C., Jeong, H., Nolan, M., Wilson, T., Tweedlie, J., Phillips, E., Senu, H., & Holland, F. (2014). The accordion and the deep bowl of spaghetti: Eight researchers' experiences of using IPA as a methodology. *The Qualitative Report*, *19*(*24*), 1–15. http://hdl.handle.net/10545/560949.

Wakely, E., & Carson, J. (2010). Historical recovery heroes: Winston Churchill. *Mental Health and Social Inclusion, 14(4)*, 36–39. doi:10.5042/mhsi.2010.0621.

Wakely, E., & Carson, J. (2011a). Historical recovery heroes: Charles Darwin. *Mental Health and Social Inclusion, 15(2)*, 66–70. doi:10.1108/20428301111140903.

Wakely, E., & Carson, J. (2011b). Historical recovery heroes: Florence Nightingale. *Mental Health and Social Inclusion, 15(1)*, 24–28. doi:10.5042/mhsi.2011.0055.

Wakely, E., & Carson, J. (2011c). Historical recovery heroes: Isaac Newton. *Mental Health and Social Inclusion, 15(3)*, 122–128. doi:10.1108/20428301111165708.

Wall, S. (2008). Easier said than done: Writing an autoethnography. *International Journal of Qualitative Methods, 7(1)*, 38–53. doi:10.1177/160940690800700103.

Ward, M., Cordle, H., Fradgley, J., & Carson, J. (2010). Recovery heroes: A profile of Matt Ward. *Mental Health and Social Inclusion, 14(1)*, 6–10. doi:10.5042/mhsi.2010.0064.

# 6 StoryTeller – Jo Mullen

*Jo Mullen and Robert Hurst*

> *Jerome:* I was first contacted by Jo in December 2017. She e-mailed me to ask if it was possible to do a PhD with the intriguing title, "From PD to PhD: An autoethnography of transformative learning." While debating the different types of PhD open to her, I opportunistically asked whether she would like to co-author a piece for my Remarkable Lives series, which she agreed to (Mullen and Carson, 2018). Remarkable Lives was aptly named. Jo more than meets the criteria for inclusion in the series. Creativity is her middle name. While she no longer works in full-time education, she spends a lot of her time coming up with highly creative resources to help people better understand personality disorder, such as "What R U like?" and her board game, "Personapoly". She was the obvious choice for this book given her creativity. She is never reluctant to offer her psychology friend advice. Of course, whether I choose to use it is a different matter, but it is always given generously.
>
> *Robert:* Jerome had spoken lots to me about Jo, and hers was one of the first names that he suggested for this project. I went in knowing little more about Jo than what I had read in her Remarkable Lives account, which I had been struck by when reading it a year earlier. I think that I got more than I bargained for! As well as being incredibly insightful, Jo was thinking about things on a conceptual level as well as a personal one. In many ways, Jo's being the first interview to be conducted was very helpful for me, as it helped me to begin shaping my foundational ideas, which were refined as the other interviews went on.

## Jo's story

For me, creativity is the foundational essence. Creativity means building, constructing, designing. And so everything is constructed or designed.

DOI: 10.4324/9781003319405-6

*Recovery*

Recovery … Now there's a big one!

In my Remarkable Lives piece, Jerome asked me about recovery. As I said, I have a problem with it in the way that it's used in a mental health sense. Because, to me, recovery suggests that there was somewhere back in the past where everything was great. So, recovery is, to me, finding some better place of health. To recover from something suggests that you've completely got over it. You've got rid of it, you've moved past it, back to full health or functioning. So I've always felt it's the wrong term to use. And you know that, because people always have to explain what it means, have to give a definition – one that might not actually explain recovery to everyone. So, if you have to do that, then surely you must realise the term is wrong. So, in a way, if you label things, you limit it to either *your* understanding, or a common understanding. And, I just think with recovery, it's caused unnecessary confusion.

I don't think it's even trying to generalise something that's a lot more personal – I just think they're idiots – whoever's decided that this is the term to base a whole movement around, and put a whole lot of money into. It's not good for people who already have low self-esteem, because if they take the common meaning – which is to get over something completely – they might think "oh, well … I'm never gonna be able to do that". So, already, they're excluded. And, there are some people I know who've been very unwell, and they wouldn't even be able to articulate anything about recovery. It's just not in their here-and-now.

Some people are so acutely distressed that they're not able to even see that that's how they are. So I think it's, I hate to use the term, just another neoliberal strategy. I've been guilty of this myself, of creating neat models, like CHIME is. But I feel strongly that everybody should be facilitated to create their own model. Whether it is an acronym, or a diagram, or an image. For me, there's always a power imbalance if somebody says, "here's a model, I'm gonna help you through it". Now, they might have a chance to say, "these are my goals", but you're still imposing something on them by saying "well, do it within this model" – CHIME, PERMA, whatever. One, I think it's wrong morally. But also, I don't see how that can work. In a whole range of situations, a change can only be successful if it's been initiated by that person or that group. You need to feel ownership of something to feel motivated to create that change.

Even the word "empowerment". It's been used as something that you do *to* people. "We will help to empower this person". Well, again, if people aren't aware, if you try to empower someone, it will be *your* definition of empowerment. *Your* standard, *your* goals.

I don't think most people are brave enough, yet, to actually sit with people. To be their loving witness without trying to steer them anywhere. The one reason why a lot of services fail, and people delivering services get demoralised, is because they don't have a higher perspective. With how I live my life, I know that whatever happens to me physically or emotionally, I'm safe. So, I can be with somebody who is in deep distress, and I don't think, "I've got to save them, I've got to do this, this, or this", because that's *my* agenda. I'm not saying I would wish to allow someone to die, I'd probably just dive in if someone was gonna do that. But, if you start from a place of allowing someone to express themselves, whatever they're feeling, in whatever way, that is what is beneficial. When you think in your head, "oh, I wonder how I can get them to change to that, or that", you're not actually giving them full respect.

Looking from a higher perspective, how arrogant of me to think that I know what that person set as their learning objectives for this incarnation, now! I might actually be interfering with their process if I have not been invited. If I thought "oh, I must step in here, I must do this, I must do that" without being invited, then that is immediately disempowering. Because it's not to do with them. It's to do with my unease at what I'm witnessing and what they're going through. So, I think I'm very wary of terminology, of models, when they're applied to people. I'm all for encouraging people to create their own way of operating; using personal "models" is the only pure way of operating, I think.

So, is there a better word than "recovery"? You don't even have to call it anything. Because as soon as you call something "something", everybody, whether it's one individual or a group, will have an idea of what that means to them, based on their own experiences. So, it's better not to actually try to contain any experience within a word or a phrase or a model. And if you think about it, we do not have the right to do that with other people.

Everybody has the capacity to steer their own path. As I say, if somebody asks for support and you're able to give it, and you feel comfortable about giving it – that's different. But what you can do instead, is if they haven't asked, you can sit with them, you can just witness, you can talk to them. That's not intruding. That's my view, anyway.

### CHIME

When I was a columnist for the journal *Mental Health and Social Inclusion*, the title I chose was, "Chronicles of one woman's journey towards wellbeing". Now, you're only allowed 8 words in the title, so that's 7. So, every time I put a colon after it, and every edition, every issue, I put one word. So, one was "connectedness", another one was "identity". I've used that because as somebody said to me – "If you can walk on water, take the boat". Which means, if you know who you are and how you want to live, then you're not threatened by someone else's journey or belief system.

I would happily go into a church, or a mosque, or whatever … I'd probably draw the line at Tory Party HQ, actually! But you see what I'm getting at. So for me, if other people use that recovery model and they find it helpful, it's not a problem for me. But I'm speaking to you in a way that I wouldn't speak to somebody about it if they were in distress, because if they'd chosen that, I'm not gonna interfere. I'm just saying that the problem for me is that somebody has decided on this model in an ego-driven way. It's fine if they came up with CHIME for themselves, and then other people saw it and said, "that might help me", but I suspect that wasn't the case. I suspect that whoever put that together thought (this sounds awful, but it's not meant to), "oh, I think that this would help *loads* of people". And you don't know that, and you shouldn't ever assume that. And then suddenly, it's become this big giant kind of bible. And that's a worry in any sphere of life. Because it can make people feel that they're obliged to use it, and that if they can't for some reason, or it doesn't resonate with them, there's perhaps something wrong with them. All of us have the potential to feel that in lots of ways throughout our lives, and you don't need another opportunity to feel that.

I think it might be better to move past the CHIME thing – protect yourself as much as you can, Robert! We'll say at the end of this – "No interviewers were harmed in the making of this chapter!".

### *Creativity*

It means the capacity to build something new. That doesn't always mean from scratch. For me, in a lot of ways, it means taking something from here, and something from here, that may or may not have been created by a person. It might be something I've noticed. I often take components from different places and use them, maybe with a sprinkle of something else (usually from up above), to present something in a different way. And I would say that to present something in a different way can refer to physical objects, ideas, concepts, art – anything – words, stories … it's anything that's new.

I'm so grateful that I've got to the stage where I see creativity as a natural part of me. I often have lots of projects on the go, and not all of them go anywhere. But that's ok because the joy, for me, is in the creation. And often I've said to people, "take this idea, you can have it, I'm not charging – if it's useful, do something with it".

Creativity, for me, is obviously – and I emphasise that word – is *obviously* an essential force of, and within, our universe. Creation is going on the whole time. Whether it's a plant growing another petal, or us finding a new path in the woods. Every single thing is creating, and every moment is completely new. We do like to look back at our past, and see patterns, but that's only one way of looking at it – you can also look at different events, even though they're similar, as completely discreet. For me, something – whether it's an essence or a form or an idea – is created in every nanosecond. You can't put a number on those infinite, tiniest moments.

The essence of something is, I would say, the intention. So, *all* of what it seeks to be, or ought to become, perhaps. And you have to be clear; the essence could be a quality, like kindness. Or, it could be strength, like that of a tree, or it could be like the fluidity of a river. But, as I say, you've got the essence, and then you've got the form. The form is flexible, the essence is set. But you can manifest the form that you wish from that essence.

You're gonna have to go for a lie down after this, aren't you?!

### *Creativity on the journey*

I would say it *is* me. Creativity is the way I speak, the way I express myself, the way I feel; it is the very essence of me. So, anything that comes out of me, has been created. Whether it's a word, a whisper, a movement. I've created that, and it's come from me. Over the years, I've used my creativity in visual form and in written form to express myself. I've used creative non-fiction, I've used posters to explain things. It's that which I make, whether physical or digital, that is an extension of me. It's not a separation from me, my whole being is in that creation, because there's no separation between me and an artifact that has come from me.

I wouldn't even say my creations are an extension of my internal self. They *are* me. They are me represented in a different form. The stories I've written, the posters I've designed... human beings will see that as a separation – this is an object, this is a person. But actually, there's no boundaries. These boundaries are artificial. They're an illusion. But we have them to help people to discern and to understand. So, as I said, everything that I have created in a physical form *is* me.

### *Creativity as communication tool*

It can be a bit like a communication device, a Rosetta Stone, maybe. But certainly nowadays, I feel that it's not my business how other people interpret what I put out. Some things I suspect might be helpful for some people, and some people have told me as much. But that shouldn't be my reason for creating it. I create because I create. I am because I am. If people can resonate with that and find it useful, then that's great. But as I've said to you before, I try to live from a place of service now; I don't mean that in the way of, "I'm creating this because it would be good for X, Y, and Z", because that's arrogant, and that's me putting my assumptions onto them.

All I can do is create from the urges I get to produce whatever I produce. And then, if I share them with other people, it's then not my business what they do with it. I know that sounds a bit harsh, but I think sometimes you have to be pure about these things.

### *Helping with creativity*

It's like a moral code. I think if you've ever done a counselling course, or whatever, if your intention and reason for doing a counselling course or training as a therapist is to help people, then you're in the wrong place. Creativity comes into this in what we produce, because the only way to serve, as a way to end suffering, is to facilitate someone else's journey. But based on *their* terms. And again, as I said, if they find what you produce or what you say or how you support them useful, great. And if they don't, that's great too.

What I've learned over the years is that I was deluding myself for a long time, thinking I was helping people when, in fact, the reality was I was probably doing more interfering than helping. So again, labelling things is dangerous because you can say, "oh, well, I was only helping", and it will discourage you from actually looking at what you've done – because it was helping, right? "I didn't do any damage, because I was helping". *Now* what I do, is if people ask for my help, if I can give it, and I feel that I can give it in a good way, I'll say yes. If can't, I'll say no.

And if I *do* see a friend in need or whatever, and I know that I have something that I could offer that might help, I only offer once. If I offer more than once, then that's about me, and not about them; my need to say, "well actually, I've got the solution". So, there's nothing wrong with saying to people "well, how about this?". But you're stepping over the line if you keep insisting.

### Form of creativity

This essence of creativity, I don't really channel it in any way. I allow it to take whatever form it takes, at whatever time. Again, no restrictions, because then you're open to any possibility, and that's exciting. We as humans, we will always put things into categories and create systems. But that's because we're afraid of *not knowing*; we need to try to pin everything down for certain, and that's what the pandemic has shown. Before the pandemic, if you book a holiday in a few months' time, it's gonna happen. But actually – in reality – there's no certainty that you'll go on that holiday, as was the case even before the pandemic! It's been an illusion we have created. All of these pseudo-certainties, if you like, because we're too afraid of not knowing what the next step might be. But it's only in that not knowing, of feeling comfortable in not knowing, that the real power of our own innate creativity can be at its best.

Creativity links in with that existential unknown – it must – because we can't create what's natural to us if we have limitations.

### Creative process

It's natural, as I said, it's *me*… being myself. I feel free to be myself. Everything I create and do is inspired. And that feels good to me because I'm connected to the source of all creativity. Creativity is the most important, or *the* all-encompassing force, of the universe.

If you think about how we grow up and we're told we have to fit into this model of rules, or this group of societal expectations… we're being *squeezed* all the time. It doesn't matter whether you're politically on the left or the right; it's imposed. If something is imposed on you, it means it's not natural for you. Because if it were natural for you, you would naturally go in that direction. But it's all ok because we we're here to learn about ourselves. And, as I said, everything is an opportunity to learn if you wish to see it that way.

### Creativity as means of learning about the self

They are one and the same. Everything I've written, everything I have produced, has been as a result of something new that I've discovered about myself. Or why, as I said, I try to communicate something, like my road map – feeling anxious about attending a hospital appointment; I looked at making it into stages of where I first received the letter, and then a week before, the night before, all of that. So it's about learning, and you can't actually separate the two. The process evolving and my creative outputs, they are one and the same. They are just different manifestations of the same thing.

I use the word "artifacts" – each thing I create is an artifact in a museum that details my development. And it's my own museum, of course. Anybody can have their own museum. Yes, I actually put things in order. But it wouldn't just be by date, it would mark my evolutionary process – like eras. All of my creative outputs represent a stage further on my journey to… well I suppose to use Maslow's term, "self-actualisation". But it's a combination of personal development and spiritual development. It's becoming more *who I am*. It makes sense that it's the essence of creativity that has driven my evolution.

But even better, isn't it, if we can harness that – if we can take charge of how we express our own creativity. On our own journey of evolution, we can choose to use our creativity for good or for bad. And that's where people talk about "fate". Well, yes, we come in with a blueprint, but we also have free will. So, we can have like, an overall idea of where we're going but you can choose the path, you can choose how to get there – that's not preordained.

### Artistic vs creative

Is there a difference between creativity and artistic-ness? … No. As I said, you know … being artistic, if you mean painting or sculpting, that's just one way of expressing creativity.

Sculpture is a form of creativity; painting is a form of creativity. You can have one central essence, but it can take many forms. And that's something that we need to learn, as a human race. That we all come from the same place, and we all express that same place or places or essence – which I feel is creativity – in different ways. But some people feel they have the right to say, "I don't think you should express creativity like that". And going back to what some people say is mental illness – who is to decide whether someone's experience is right or wrong? It comes back to that need to know, that need to be certain. "I need to know what box to put that in, especially when I feel threatened by it, or I haven't experienced it myself".

There are over seven billion sparks of the divine on this planet, and I'm sure they all see things – the art world as you say – in different ways.

An art critic scoring a painting, to me that's exactly the same as the recovery models. It's giving everything a score. In a way it's the journey versus the destination, isn't it? If you grade something, like a piece of artwork, you're looking at the destination; you're looking for a final point. To say, "right, that's it, it's done". No, it's been criticised, it's been judged. But again (you'll probably get fed up of me saying it) that limits it. It won't let it go anywhere else. And more importantly, it won't let any*one* else come in and offer a different interpretation.

The person who created it will have their own interpretation. But, if they were really really precious about that, if it was like, "the only interpretation", then we'd never put it in the gallery, show it off or anything. You have to feel comfortable with being vulnerable, to allow people to see different things in it to what you see or what you intend. The word "sharing" is in my head – Do you really want to share? Allowing anybody to interpret something whatever way they wish? Or is it a conditional sharing – that you see things from my point of view, or that you give me praise for it?

To share properly and unconditionally requires vulnerability. But many people don't think about what their intention is. They might just use the word "share", without thinking about what they expect back. So, if you share for the sake of sharing, unconditionally, then you allow people to make use of whatever you've created, in whichever way they feel will help them, or mean something to them. But if you're only putting something out and saying, "right, this is what it means, no one had dare criticise it or try to reinterpret it", there's then a difference.

And you know what, even *those* things, you can't say are right or wrong. But I think it's always helpful, for your own personal development, to know why you're doing something. In the simplest terms, "what am I looking for here? Am I sharing my creativity in the way I express it just because it's a natural part of me? Because I can't help it?" Just as I said, a flower can't help growing. It doesn't limit itself. It doesn't say, "I'm only prepared to grow this much" or whatever. "If you want me to grow more, you have to tell me the most amazing jokes and I might grow another couple of centimetres". They don't put any conditions on it. They grow because it's natural, they don't question it. They don't question things like we do. We're more used to, or conditioned, to limiting ourselves – our natural abilities or essence – than we are to allowing it to develop organically in ways that feel natural to us, to not constrain ourselves.

### *Nature of creativity*

The force that is the same as creativity, and this is where it gets a bit mushy if you don't like these things, is love. Love is the creative force of the universe. The two are the same. It's love that is unconditional. It's like emptying a big box of Lego onto the world, and saying – "Right, there aren't any sets here, you can just make whatever you want, whatever resonates, go and pick that up and build".

Creation is an act of love because you are sharing yourself unconditionally. If you're doing that with people, you are showing them love, because it's saying, "here's my offering, but I'm not telling you what you should do with it, or even if you should accept it". Cause the problem is, love has been misappropriated by the big, organised religions. You know, you can only express love if it's in this way or this way or this way. Well, that's not freedom, is it? That's not natural. That's not creative.

And some people, they like that. But for me, I have never joined a religion, or a political party, because once you sign up to a set of rules or guidance, you put yourself in a bit of a conundrum. There's bound to be something along the way that you perhaps think, "I don't feel quite right about that". So, do you then carry on being part of the tribe, or do you actually decide to leave the tribe, because you are putting your own morals first? I would rather have the freedom to check in with myself, to make my own decisions based on what I think is right, rather than hand all responsibility for that moral or political decision-making over to some other entity. For me, in a way, if you commit yourself to a group, that's got a dogma, or a set of rules, you're saying, "I no longer have to take responsibility for what I feel is right"; you're giving that up. Whereas, creating harnesses that energy, and being creative is the ultimate freedom. And, as I said, with it, hopefully comes awareness, and personal responsibility. To be creative is a channelling of that responsibility, having awareness and putting it out there. It's all interlinked.

I would say it's like ... you know how people like to do Venn diagrams? Well, the problem for me is that, it does show links between things, but it's very static isn't it? And I think, say if you've got things like responsibility and creativity and self-awareness. Well ... they're more like that slime stuff that's popular. You know, it's kind of like they morph into each other. Sometimes this one's a bit bigger, and sometimes it's this one that's bigger; you have to allow things to move and change.

Things can't be static. As soon as you've created something, be prepared for it to change. Otherwise, how can we move on? How can we move anywhere if we stand still?

An artifact you create might be an expression of one moment in time, but as you move forward, it is your relationship to it, and understanding of it, that will change and morph.

Let's make it topical. You take an artifact, like a statue of a slave trader, and it's not until somebody looks at it anew and says, "hang on a minute! Why are we celebrating this person with a statue when we don't feel quite comfortable about it?". And what they did with the Edward Colston statue in Bristol was, they responded. People responded from their feelings. It wasn't an academic argument that pushed "him" into the river, was it? It was people's feelings. They were looking at this statue that they probably walked past all their lives – and suddenly, they're looking at it in a new light, from a different perspective. You can't force feelings. It was just looking at it in a different way and going, "God, that's bad ... . Get him in the canal!".

It was only afterwards that the people perhaps who didn't like it happening were starting to create a big argument as to why they shouldn't have done it. But it wasn't planned. People just suddenly realised, "Oh! This has been here *all* my life, it's not appropriate, get a big anchor, get it in the canal."

That was creative.

The people created a different narrative about that bit of metal. That's all it is, a bit of metal, isn't it? Let's face it. On a stone plinth. It shows how much meaning we ascribe to these things.

I mean, look at Mondrian as a painter. He's got different coloured squares, and a six-year-old child might come along and say, "oh, I can do that!". And people will go, "no, no, it's Mondrian, it's different from yours!". So, it's not the technique or the thing itself, but what people see in it.

### Creations of others

For the first day of secondary school, we had art in the afternoon, and it was art history. I loved it, learning some of the meanings behind things and symbols. I love symbols. And so, if somebody has created some artwork, I really do like to know why they created it, why they shaped it in the way they did. I'm interested to know how they are using whatever medium to express themselves.

And I just love architecture. Again, because it's so imbued with meaning and symbolism. For example you've got the Bank of England. It's created and designed in a neo-classical style in order to say, "this is reminiscent of Ancient Greece; this is a building to be respected, and trusted … because it's old, it's really old".

And then you've got the green building revolution, where comfort is prioritised, but it's not decadent. I do like design programmes on TV, but there was one that started with Tiny Tempah fronting it. Now, I like him, but I couldn't cope with the subject matter because he was looking at people who have designed houses for themselves that are massive, decadent. It just didn't sit right with me – the prices of houses now, people not able to eat or live in a home. I just couldn't watch it. So, in a way, if I *had* watched it, I would have seen those creations as ugly, even though they weren't designed to be ugly. For me, I put a moral interpretation on what they were designing and building.

It's not all about aesthetics, but other people's intentions behind it. There are also people within the mental health arena who, like Dolly Sen, use humour and sarcasm and wit to basically take the piss – she uses her artwork to do that, and good on her. There's poetry too, and of course posters have often had an anti-establishment or challenging aspect to them. Record covers. People coming from a certain perspective, and I think a lot of powerful messaging has been put across and adopted by people because it's been embedded in art, whether that's a poster, or an object, poetry …

We imbue our creations with meaning of our own, and then let others see what they see. That's all we can do. But it's also what we owe to ourselves. Until we feel comfortable and secure in feeling like that is our birth right, then people are suppressed. Their creativity, which I feel is our natural essence, is suppressed.

Things shouldn't have to fit a certain style, cause that's a way of constraining what I feel is natural. If my natural creativity hadn't been suppressed from an early age, my life journey would have been very different. Possibly not as adventurous and as exciting as I've had. I've got there in the end, and as I say, it's fascinating to look back. To see how I've gone from one step to another, and now feeling confident about expressing myself in all sorts of ways, creatively.

The stifling of that creativity caused a lot of difficulties. And the problem is criticism, isn't it? From all angles of life. You show a bit of yourself, and this goes for everybody, whether people have experienced any form of obvious abuse or not …

we all hear from the outside, whether from our caregivers or society or newspapers or whatever, that if there's something that we're doing or expressing, a big voice comes and says, "No! You don't do it like *that*". They might say it in a nice way, but it's still saying, "what you're doing is not the right way". And so, you're automatically turned away from your natural path that you're on. It just takes the life out of you, and once you're aware of this process, it's a lifetime of getting yourself back onto that original path – obviously now with the whole lifetime of experiences – but you're essentially returning to your Self, with a capital S.

So, what you might call "recovery" is in many ways a reclaiming of those creative essences. A way of discovering the Self through creativity. Actually, "reclaiming" would be a better word than "recovery", because I believe that when we struggle, if we have conflicts within ourselves, it's because we're not being allowed, or allowing ourselves, to be who we essentially are. There's something a bit off. So, for me, "reclaiming" my true self and expressing that through my core essence of creativity is where I want to be.

### *Everyday creativity*

OK. You got a pen? Right, OK then. Posters, presenting, delivering training sessions. Writing short stories, writing creative non-fiction, as a columnist. What else do I do? I like using a play on words for almost everything, in every conversation. I love manipulating words to produce different meanings. I like looking at words and seeing what's hidden behind them, whether they're anagrams, or taking bits out, whatever, and relating them to other things – connecting different concepts or ideas or words to things that are meaningful to me. That's creative because it's building. It's building my own philosophy if you like. And as I said, I am a magician. I can make things happen. I'm good at manifesting.

> *Robert:* At times, I felt as though Jo was challenging me, pushing me to see things differently. I appreciated this. I was inspired by her description of creativity as an essence, a different form of Self more than just an extension. How it can be the ultimate form of expression and freedom. Seen this way, creativity is vital. It is the form in which we can express our true Selves.

### Reference

Mullen, J., & Carson, J. (2018) Remarkable lives: Jo Mullen in conversation with Jerome Carson. *Mental Health and Social Inclusion*, *22*(3), 121–127. doi:10.1108/MHSI-03-2018-0013.

# 7    StoryTeller – Michelle McNary

*Michelle McNary and Robert Hurst*

| | |
|---|---|
| *Jerome:* | Of the three people I introduced to Robert for this book, Michelle was the person I met first. I had been asked to see Michelle when I worked as a clinical psychologist in the community. There was no doubt that Michelle was a very creative person. Her story of her own mental health problems was told in two chapters in books that I co-edited on mental health recovery stories (Cordle et al., 2011; Davies et al., 2011). Michelle became a key person in the Recovery Group that I established in the South-West Lambeth service, and it was some time after this that we came up with the idea of making a film about recovery (Carson et al., 2012). |
| | Initially, Michelle wanted to make this about her own journey, but in the end, we decided it might be easier if she looked at the recovery journey of others. Dr Paul Wolfson auditioned potential participants with Michelle. They decided who they would select. I was equally sure to play no role whatsoever in how the film was to be made. That was to be the creative direction of Michelle with some advice from Paul. In the end they selected four people, Dolly, Ben, Gordon and James. |
| | The resulting film presented the four of them as "philosophers of recovery" and has been viewed over 21,000 times on YouTube (Maudsley NHS, 2010). Michele's creativity shines through in this film. My relationship, initially as her therapist, became as a co-producer of recovery initiatives and much more of a partnership. I suggested we ask Michelle to participate in this project as she was a highly creative individual. If she never makes another film, this will be enough to secure her legacy. She was shortlisted for a Mind Media Award, which went to Ruby Wax. I know who should have really been given that Award. |
| *Robert:* | Having been a student of Jerome's, I saw Michelle's *Recovery* film more than once. It was clear to all of the student cohort how |

DOI: 10.4324/9781003319405-7

> rightfully proud Jerome was for having played his part in getting this film made. Michelle's name was one we heard a lot. As such, I was somewhat nervous to meet her. I needn't have worried. Michelle was incredibly polite, kind and insightful. But enough from me – we have framed our shot, now let us pan the camera around to Michelle.

**Michelle's story**

I think it's something in me. I'm not sure about everyone else, but something within me drove towards creativity, because it gave me some sort of comfort. It's kind of like a hunger for me, making films. Creativity is something so private, and yet also something that can touch the lives of so many people.

*Recovery*

Oh, recovery. Recovery. God, that's so hard to explain. I'll have to take my time.

In a sense, you want to be "well" with recovery. But I think there's stages. When you first come out of hospital, you're just glad to get out of hospital. Then you have to get back into real life. And then you have to live *with* a mental illness. Recovery, I'd say … what would I say? … Do you know Patricia Deegan? Now, she's someone that I was really interested to read about, and she inspired me to get more well.

I really worked at recovery, it wasn't something that happened overnight. It took weeks, years, to get better at it. But I don't think you can cure mental illness. Well maybe let's not call it mental illness, I don't know what you call it … mental distress? Taking medication, that's part of recovery, because if you don't take medication, in my opinion, you're not going to be as well as you can be, because you're gonna have the symptoms. Even when the side effects are as bad as they are, I'm not sure how recovered I would be if I wasn't on medication and not having talking therapy. I used to go to meetings at SLaM (South London and Maudsley), and the Mosaic Clubhouse. Stuff like that, where you meet other people, and you make friends who you can talk to about your recovery, it helps. I began speaking to Jerome about my mental health, and as I said I had a lot of talking therapy working on myself and my goals and aspirations that I have for myself. So recovery is a journey, not a destination. Do you know what I mean? It's a long process, not just an ending point. It's about trying to get to the best place that you can at that moment in time.

But you've got to know your limitations as well. Because sometimes I expect a bit too much and I forget I'm mentally unwell, and other people forget that I'm mentally unwell cause I come across so well. And I *am* well, but I still have symptoms. Like today, I don't know why, I was anxious, and I'm like "well what's that about?". It's not very nice, because you feel that you're not in control of yourself. I think that's the thing about recovery – the more recovered you are, the more you believe in yourself. It gives you that feeling of being in control.

And also what I think is really important about recovery is all the people around you. Your family and all your friends. I mean, I probably wouldn't have gotten this far without help from my family and friends, you know? I appreciate that.

The thing is, and I think Dolly Sen says it in my *Recovery* film – recovery is different to everyone. Everyone's got their unique journey along the way. By being in collaboration, like I was with my *Wellbeing* film (which isn't about recovery, but it is still about wellbeing, and recovery *is* wellbeing) and getting yourself out there, you find there are other people out there that can help you. So if you are depressed, there *is* someone to speak to, and I think that's a brilliant resource for everyone.

## *CHIME*

### *Connectedness*

I think connectedness is good. Because what can happen with people who have mental distress is becoming quite isolated with your problems. I think I have that, to a degree. I like to have a routine. I'm not good at just doing things spontaneously like I used to, which I find a big change … I'm different like that, I'm a bit more cautious than I used to be. I don't know why that is, but when I turned 50, I know it's just a number, but I felt like… what have I achieved? What have I done? I've spent so many years with this film thing, and I haven't done all the other things that I wanna do. And you get regrets and stuff like that. Then I had to say to myself "listen, you're 50 years old, look how far you've come, considering" … I mean I left school with no qualifications. I was very mentally ill at school, so I couldn't cope with the pressure of my qualifications and stuff like that.

### *Hope*

Hope. Oh my goodness, see that's the crux of it. If you don't have hope …

I have been hopeless. Like Patricia Deegan said, it can happen when you are unwell … and it is awful. But you have to dig deep and find some hope, and have a positive outlook. It's very important. To not let mental illness stop you from getting happiness. Or, for example I wanna try and go back into photography again, but I'm worrying whether I'm good enough. That I think is part of my mental illness … "Am I good enough?", that was always there … and I don't think that will ever leave me.

Hope is what pulls you through, makes you give it a go.

### *Identity*

I haven't got a problem with telling people about my mental distress. But they seem to get embarrassed, or they kind of don't really understand what it's about. Sometimes people can be cruel. I was at a party with this guy, and we were talking, and it came up that I was mentally ill, he said "oh, everyone's mentally ill". And so I asked, "Have you been hospitalised? Have you had ECT treatment? Do you have ongoing therapy? Do you take medication?" "No", he said. "Well you're talking a load of bollocks then" – excuse my language. After that he got nasty, called me a "psycho bitch". So that's a part of identity when you have a mental health diagnosis. There is absolutely stigma.

Identity is being yourself as well, and not to be scared to delve in. Even with recovery, it's difficult to get yourself out there. But if you don't, a lot of people get depressed. Or, for me, if I'm like that, if I'm depressed, I'll eat, or I'll drink too much, I'll self-medicate. So I have to try and keep some sort of routine. Not 100%, I'm a very flexible person, but I have a routine. So to be honest with you, I don't like to mix 100% with people with mental health issues. I find it very stressful. Because I'm a good listener normally, and people open up to me for some reason. And I do actually find that quite difficult. Dealing with my own mental stress, and the reasons why I became mentally ill, and I actually believe that started as a child if I look back. But it's awful when you're in that hopelessness stage, or you don't think it's worth it. And I know that I was talking to Dolly, and she said she's lost a lot of friends through suicide. And I have felt like that. I don't think that's to do with identity, I'm veering off again!

*Meaning*

I think that's important. If you do meaningful things, like therapeutic things, it's really good for recovery. I'll go swimming. I've been swimming this morning, because I knew I needed to be chilled out when I spoke to Robert! And I feel quite comfortable now, so it worked. But meaning, God, you can look at that as a philosophical question. You can look at that as what life means to you or to other people around you. For me, meaning is … living. Not living the dream, necessarily, it's … It's so vast.

Do we have a purpose? Are we just on this earth to procreate?

You know what's really interesting? Just saying about meaning. I'm reading this book called *Origins*, I don't know if you've heard about it. It's really good, and it's all about how the earth shaped human life and not the other way round. Like how we evolved over time and stuff like that. That's quite interesting for me. And that kind of gives me meaning to the world. I love to read. So I read quite a few books. And if I do read, the problem is if I do read, I don't do anything else. I sit there with a cup of tea and a vape and just go. But I do find reading a therapeutic activity. Very, very helpful.

So you have to give your own life meaning. Everyone deserves a meaningful life. And I think Gordon McManus said that, didn't he? In the *Recovery* film.

*Empowerment*

Swimming today gave me empowerment, actually. Made me feel strong, on a physical level.

People need to be proactive, they really do. And you know what, I do a little project with Vocation Matters, down in Brixton. And we did an "expanding your world" activity. We had about 10 people for 5 weeks. We'd start off with showing the *Wellbeing* film, and then we would go into groups and talk about what well-being means to them, stuff like that. Now that, that gave me a sense of purpose and empowerment. It was sharing my story, and others can take stuff from me, hopefully. I am a good role model to some people, and people will see the *Recovery* and *Wellbeing* films and think "that girl, she's going through it. She understands. She's empathetic about, and sensitive to other people's distress".

Sharing my story is a big part of my purpose and my empowerment. And my family, of course, and friends. Definitely. It's a scary thing when you put yourself out there. I don't know about you, Robert. To be scrutinised. I am so hard on myself. If someone told me they didn't like my film, I'd probably be quite hurt. However, I would prefer the truth.

### *Creativity*

You know what, the problem is, right … I was mentally ill, and I was undiagnosed as a child. I remember always feeling different. I was bullied at school because everyone thought I was a weirdo and stuff like that. And I never used to think the same way as everyone else did. So what I did was, I found ways of not ignoring it, but putting it aside.

I used to do a lot of gymnastics, and I felt that gave me a sense of freedom. I didn't feel trapped in this body. I felt that I was free like the wind, and I think that's creativity.

You're looking for meaning and purpose, you're searching. You're open. For me, I'm very open to ideas, and to interesting people. Like Jerome for example. I'd never met anyone quite like him. And, you know, he's just so good at what he does. And he's so different than a lot of the other ones (you can tell Jerome that I've given him some good PR!).

It comes in so many forms, doesn't it, creativity? My mum's very creative. My great grandma was a painter. My dad did acting. My brother did acting, and we both ended up going to film school. That was my biggest goal – to go to Bournemouth film school. And that's where I found my creative voice, really. Because I was making art films before that, but then I got chance to make some 15-minute dramas and things.

When I spoke to Jerome, I hadn't made films for a while. And I didn't see that coming, *Recovery*. I just didn't see it coming. I thought I'd never make films again. Cause I didn't fit into the demographic. I was too old. I didn't have any contacts. I had no money. I was still thinking "I wanna be a filmmaker". And that actually, my creativity, was making me feel even worse. Because there was that drive, but I was also unwell. I was paranoid, I thought people were reading my mind. Not hallucinations, that happened in hospital, but part of creativity is a kind of madness, and a sense of chaos. And I think it is this coming out of that and making it meaningful.

### Caution in creativity

With creativity, be careful if you've got mental health issues. That's my thing. Make sure that when you do it, you're in the right place mentally. Cause I'm thinking of making my film *Climbing Walls*. It's a three-part drama. My beginning, middle, and end. So it's the beginning of where it all started, then being mentally ill, and finally recovery. I raised money to make it, but I wasn't ready at the time. So that might be my goal in the future. But if that is the case, I wanna work with another writer and probably won't direct it myself. Because of stress. And I find it very difficult … when I'm creative, sometimes it makes me anxious. I dunno if you've heard that before. Other people get lost in the whole thing, and they don't look at it like that, but I do, unfortunately. I have to protect myself; I have to be careful not to get unwell over it.

In that creative zone, you've gotta be cautious. Like I've just tried to learn guitar, and I'm finding it really stressful. So I've stopped. I don't understand why I can't just go and play a guitar. My mum was like, "Don't worry, you're not doing it for an award. Just do it."

### Being creative versus being artistic

I'll say my boyfriend was an "artist", he was artistic. But it's all creating something, isn't it? He was making 2D animation, and he did a short film, and he was artistic … I mean I can't draw for love nor money. But I'm creative, I find creativity in anything. Like I say about my mum – she got a new place, and she started to buy things on the internet. We designed the way her house would be. And that gives her real pleasure, and that's what I miss. To get just that pleasure as well.

For me, I find it very stressful to be creative again because I'm scared that the creativity will take me to places that are difficult. Do you understand what I mean by that? I did creativity when I was a kid because it was an escape thing. Because I was bullied and that, I was told I was a weirdo and stuff, so I found creativity a comfort. It was my little thing that no one could touch. My private thing, where nobody could tell me what to do. I was empowered to do it myself.

### Distress and creativity

Mentally distressed people go through such horrible experiences. With the hallucinations, and being totally out of control. I think that is the worst thing. And these things that are coming into your mind – where are they coming from? Is it reality?

I think if you're creative, you're more prone to it as well. Cause you look at Van Gogh, and I know this is a bit of a cliché, but look at all the artists – emotional wrecks. I'm sure that Van Gogh would have liked some clozapine or something! To cheer him up! Could take a Prozac. I'm on fluoxetine, and I take vitamin D, for example. All these little things all add up to make you feel better.

Recovery needs to be holistic. You can do yoga and meditation, too. I think anyone can do that to make themselves more well. It's not just people who are mentally ill. But I think mentally ill people deserve to get some happiness and some comfort.

### How creativity has helped

It brought me out of my mental distress. I got the most pleasure out of editing *Recovery*. I could be totally creative there, doing what I call the cut-and-paste method. The way that my film is. And I have used a lot of other people's material because of that. And I got that from the writer William Burroughs. He said that he did a cut-and-paste method on his books. So what he'd do, he'd write things down on bits of paper, and just put them together, jumbled together and thought "what am I gonna create out of all these different ideas?".

So my film was a cut-and-paste, and also it's very unique. I think also it's like a docu-drama. It's a documentary, but there's bits in it that are dramatic, because I come from a drama background. So I wouldn't say it was a documentary per se, but as I say, *Recovery*, when I was editing, I used to sit there for 12 hours a day. I absolutely loved it. I might even go back to editing, we'll see.

It gave me a real focus. I felt I was achieving something. And a friend said to me "you know what Michelle", she said, "whatever happens, you've got a legacy". You know, and there's that aspect to it as well, which I thought was a really nice way of saying it. That your creativity is unique, and you've got a voice, express it. I like that word "legacy". I made something that came from within me, and put it out there, and it will stay out there.

### Sharing something of yourself through creativity

It's important to share, as scary as it is. I've done all these different talks to people, and I was absolutely terrified. Jerome's saying "Michelle, talk about *you*", but it's so hard to look at your stuff and be introspective. Because you are so... well, I am quite critical of my stuff, and I'm sure other creative people are. You can always do better. The problem with creativity is sometimes the outcome is not what you thought it would be. That is where the frustration with me starts. Can I get what's going on in my head, onto the film? And if I don't, I'm always looking for the next one. It's a bit like a drug in a sense, you know? You're looking for the most perfect film you can. Chasing a high.

You're constantly trying to learn from that one, to do the next one. It's like I said to you about *Recovery* and *Wellbeing*. I think *Wellbeing* is better than *Recovery*. But then I learnt from that. I was disappointed about *Recovery*, person-ally. Because I didn't get enough cutaways, I had to do the cut-and-paste method. But I didn't want to do the same as everyone else. I wanted to make it unique. And it is unique.

### Creative process

There are idiosyncrasies, almost. I think creative people are quite eccentric, as well. Method-wise, what I do is that once I've had a few beers, I get on the computer and just type a load of old rubbish I think. And then I look at it and I think "ahh that's not actually too bad". Because at the moment, as I say, I'm trying to promote my *Climbing Walls* drama. So I'm on that at the moment, and I just do it when I feel like it. Years ago, when I was like really really into filmmaking, I mean that was my *sole* purpose, I would sit there for hours and hours and hours and read books and theory of films. And also worked as a teacher as well. I had this drive.

As a teacher, that was that. And then the process, as I say, it's quite random for me. If I give myself "right, you've got till 5 o'clock", I'll stress. It's like "ohhhh I've gotta come up with this". It's … what's that word? There's a word for it, it's like the wind. It's like … how can I explain? Not inspiration. Enlightenment. Enlightenment?

I can't force it out of me anymore, but I could do. I did force it. And sometimes it is good to sit down and say that I've got from five till seven to do it. Some people are quite good at like, on the spot creativity. Like, being a director, you have to think on your feet. You do a shot list, and you have a script. So that's the way you prepare yourself to be creative. And the more that you plan it, sometimes it's good, but then you go and you do off-the-cuff stuff. I remember I was doing my short film Virago, and I thought "right, I'm gonna do a tracking shot here". And it's one of the best shots of the film. My cameraman looked at me, and I said, "I've just come up with that!", and he laughed. I just thought of it on the spot. It wasn't in the storyboard, or the script. So there you go, see – when you are being spontaneous, there isn't the same pressure.

### Creative triggers

I really like film theory. I was doing A level film theory – it was a choice between film theory and psychology, and I went with film. I was very interested in psychology as well, but I find it too hard! I'm not very academic, I don't think. But I am creative, and I am good at what I do. I'm not being a big head, I'm not like a Steven Spielberg obviously, or anyone like that. However, I do understand films. I watch films and analyse films, I love watching films. Even bad films, wondering how these directors get on, and why they've made that shot, why didn't they do that. Subtitles, too. They don't leave them on for long enough for you to read. This is all part of like, the film knowledge, general knowledge I call it.

### Consuming creativity of others

I get a lot of pleasure from creative things. Obviously watching films. But music is like… my soul. Music, for me, it's like eating and drinking. Essential. Every day I will sit for a while, just listening to music. Just to chill out. And get meaning from the records on an emotional level, understand their work. Hearing the message they're trying to communicate. Cause again they're creative aren't they, like myself. If I meet other creative people, that's lovely. We talk about stuff, and then they'll say things about my film, I think "good, that's really good that you've thought of it in that way", you know?

There is this element of sharing and community with creativity. It's no good without an audience, is it? It's no point… it's like you doing this and you're gonna do the book, you're gonna get it out there, people are gonna read all about the creativity, recovery and wellbeing, aren't they?

### Struggling with creativity

I don't have the drive like I used to, Robert. And I am questioning at the moment about this *Climbing Walls* project, I don't know … I feel I *should* do it, not necessarily that I *want* to do it. But I want people to understand the process of going through mental illness and the run up to it. It's the unique journey that I went through. If I told you about some of the hallucinations I was getting, I thought the IRA were outside my hospital door. I thought that I was gonna be hanged on a noose, and all these really crazy dreams. I thought I was in space. Mad things. And the problem is with me is that I was trying to make it cohesive, but it's so random. And I don't want people just to think "mmm, that just looks like a silly bit of film-making. It doesn't really make sense". When you create you're trying to make sense out of something that is so chaotic, put it that way.

Creativity is trying to put some structure to chaos. It's hard. Cause you do need some structure, obviously. And most people – writers, directors, whatever – they all have a process of how they work, like I said. You can't just go along on a whim.

Mind you, a guy called Fred Wiseman, he was a documentary filmmaker, he used to do things about hospitals and mental hospitals. He's done documentaries about it. What he used to, his method, was to get a camera and just leave it on for 12 hours, and just keep it ticking over. And then spend hours and days and months editing it. That's his process.

### Critiquing creativity

You can be quite harsh on people creatively. Especially… the one's that I don't like, creative people, and I was like it once – Prima donnas, a lot of them. And it's really hard to like them, but you can like their work. We're definitely of a type. A bit crazy, risk-takers. I mean I worked in offices, and my soul was … drowning. You know my creativity was like … I had to be creative, but I sort of had to work in this terrible place. But I had no money, and I had no one to really help me, I was feeling mentally ill. And I was working in these offices, and suddenly I got mentally ill. Then I met Jerome, and I did *Recovery*, so you just don't know where life's going to take you. But if you don't put yourself out there, your creativity out there, you're never gonna know.

And also about *Climbing Walls*, I can actually make my *own* decision whether to make it or not. It's empowerment, again. I feel all artists should, *must* feel that when they create something from their soul.

But the only thing with me, I always found it quite disappointing, is all. I think that's where the madness started. I became unwell. Yeah, I did. So I have to be careful about that.

### Creativity as double-edged sword

Have you met many people that are creative, where creativity makes them feel worse? Unwell? Well, I think art is, creativity is, punishing as well. Torturous. I mean, I remember being up all night for *nights* doing scripts. It's a punishing schedule that you put yourself through. And then when you get to the end, you can think "well it's not what I quite wanted". I think that's the bottom line. You have to sit back and think, what were the circumstances of that? And maybe next time you can make it better. Learn from it.

### Stifled creativity

Oh, it's terrible. I was different at school, with mental distress. That's not good. It's being in the wrong environment, I suppose isn't it? A creative environment isn't what you'll get at the office job. Temp jobs aren't gonna do it. But as I say, I'm a bit risk taker, and I followed my heart as well. I truly do have a passion for film-making. There is that as well. If you don't have that passion, and that drive, it's a very brutal business, films.

It's very hard work. People say, "creatives are lazy" and all that. That's absolute rubbish! I probably do as much as a bloody medical student in terms of studies. Reading books, thick books. Writing notes. Doing dissertations. It's not just getting out there and sticking the camera on. There's a whole way of filming. I follow certain rules, and stuff. It has a concept, if that's the word.

Creativity is a hunger. It has to be, it's never satisfied. That's the only thing. I can tell you now, every director out there, writer, whatever, is disappointed with their last past piece of work. But then you only get judged on what you did before. So I wasn't happy with *Recovery*, but I've done the *Wellbeing* film, so that for me is my goal. I got it out there and there's nothing in it that I thought I could have done better on that one. And really the weird thing is, I didn't spend nearly as much time on that as I did *Recovery*. It's weird.

It just clicked. And as I say, I was more well. I was more recovered when I did *Wellbeing*. I had learned from *Recovery*, what I didn't do, and regret doing or not doing. Again, it was a process of just coming to terms with it. And also coming to terms with being mentally ill can be a hard pill to swallow, to be honest. It's a 24-hour job, put it that way. And you *have* to take *extra* care of yourself. That's when people become unwell, when they don't look after themselves, and that's just people generally. Not just people with mental distress. If you've got that mental distress, you've got to make sure 100% that you look after yourself, and you keep yourself well.

*Creativity as sense-making*

Creativity is making sense of this, this chaos. This drive, this hunger. And you feel happy as well, sometimes with it. But over the years my creativity has changed. I think because I've worked so hard and got so mentally ill over my film, I have to be careful about creativity. I'm not sure what your other people are saying about creativity, but I was thinking about this before I even spoke to you – this life is a double-edged sword, to me. If it works for you, and you enjoy writing poetry for example and get pleasure and passion – great. I will ensure with *Climbing Walls* that I will only do it if it feels right. I have to make sure that I'm well.

On a personal note, I've got a family that is very driven. They've given me a good work ethic. My dad and my mum made us work for everything that we've got, and that in itself will help your recovery. I was in the Territorial Army for a year, and learnt a lot of skills about looking after yourself. Being disciplined about stuff, and all these things were really good. They prepared me for filmmaking – it's not that different from warfare! It's out there, it's brutal, it's hard, and it's constant. You don't get any peace. You've got people talking to you, you've got things going wrong, you've gotta think on your feet, you only got a limited time doing it.

*Risks of creativity*

When you have a dream like filmmaking and it's not realised, that hurts. Like me, I felt, before I did *Recovery*, I felt this complete … disillusionment. Maybe that's not the word … I was … heartbroken. I was heartbroken that I hadn't broken through into the industry. I went for jobs, and it never worked out. Did films, it never worked out. I tried so hard and kept pushing and pushing, and was disappointed that no one … got it. I wasn't discovered. I do follow some of the people from film school, and they're out there making films. But you know what? I don't regret it. I've got the life I've got now, I look after my mum and I'm a carer for my mum, and I absolutely love it. I do my own thing, I've got a good relationship with my mum. But the big risk, of course, is that I can get unwell. That's for *me.* I can get unwell if I look too much into myself, about my mental illness, I'm not good. I'm not good at all. Cause I'll keep repeating it, going over and over the same thing. And I won't leave it alone and it'll make me very distressed.

You've gotta find your mojo. Or whatever they call it. Find something that you're totally passionate and interested in. That is the crux of the matter with any artist, isn't it? Any creative person. If you've got the passion and a good work ethic, it's really important.

*Everyday creativity*

There is everyday creativity, like my mum. She said she was feeling a bit depressed, so I said, "go outside to your garden". And she's out there and she looks so cute. She was out there for about two hours, sorting out all her plants. And I said, "do you feel better, Mum?". She said, "yes I do". So I think you really need to know how to make yourself well, get some happiness out of it.

What about me? Cooking. Reading, as I said before, that's creative isn't it? Yoga, too. Because you are quite creative when you're doing yoga, you're doing the different poses. You know like downward dog, the cobra, stuff like that. I'm trying to be different rather than just shooting off a load of old rubbish!

I dunno, it's a curiosity that I have in life. I find everything interesting. I want to know more about it. I have that need, that searching. I think that will never stop. It just won't. I suppose we all want to know what our purpose is, but maybe that's what drives us. Maybe that's what it is.

| | |
|---|---|
| *Robert:* | Speaking to Michelle was eye-opening for me. In the process of my excitement at how beneficial creativity could be for people, I had forgotten that it is not always so. I have spent countless hours sat at a notebook trying to write, frustrated when I cannot seem to tap into any creativity. Beating myself up for not "achieving" an imagined "potential" for myself. Michelle helped bring me back down to earth in this regard – she reminded me that creativity can certainly be a double-edged sword. I also enjoyed that Michelle asked me a lot of questions – as though she was searching for answers just as much as I was … This curiosity is surely a part of her creativity, and it pushed me to keep exploring. |

## References

Carson, J., McNary, M., Wolfson, P., & Holloway, F. (2012). The making of a film about recovery. *Mental Health and Social Inclusion*, *16*(2), 72–78. doi:10.1108/20428301211232478.

Cordle, H., Fradgley, J., Carson, J., Holloway, F., & Richards, P. (Eds.) (2011). *Psychosis: Stories of recovery and hope*. Quay Books.

Davies, S., Wakely, E., Morgan, S., & Carson, J. (Eds.) (2011). *Mental health recovery heroes past and present*. Pavilion Publishing.

Maudsley NHS. (2010). Recovery and mental illness: Part one [video]. www.youtube.com/watch?v=purscrXmygc.

# 8    StoryTeller – Peter Bullimore

*Peter Bullimore and Robert Hurst*

| | |
|---|---|
| *Jerome:* | When we were looking for people to be interviewed for our book *Psychosis: Stories of Recovery and Hope* (Cordle et al., 2011), the name Peter Bullimore came up. After Hannah had interviewed Peter, I read his remarkable account. I invited him to Streatham to speak to our Recovery Group, and Peter travelled all the way down from Sheffield to South London to give a one-hour presentation on his recovery journey. He is a mesmerising speaker. Talk over, he got the train straight back to Sheffield. After I moved to Bolton, I invited him to come across and speak to our students. Again, Peter gave a memorable presentation, which was filmed (PowAnimate, 2014). Peter invited me to the Team Bullimore Christmas party at the Garrison Hotel in Sheffield, which has now become an annual event. I was fortunate to be invited to his wedding, though I am not sure that my impromptu wedding speech was welcomed by all! Peter has never been a client or patient of mine. I would like to think he sees me as a friend. I certainly value every contact I have had with him over the years. He travels all over the world empowering and educating people, has been a major figure in the Hearing Voices Network, and founded the Paranoia Network. An incredible man. His creativity can be seen in how he has able to help hundreds, maybe thousands, of people who have struggled to understand why they hear voices. He is a better trainer than I could ever hope to be. |
| *Robert:* | Again, Peter was one of those people whose story had come up time and again in Jerome's teaching. I remember being deeply moved by his account upon first reading it as an undergraduate student. Knowing Peter's international reputation, I was a touch nervous to meet him. He soon put me at ease with his wonderful Yorkshire sense of humour and thorough honesty. |

DOI: 10.4324/9781003319405-8

## Peter's story

If you think about Van Gogh – he had to stop drinking a little bit, or he couldn't paint as well. It's a really heavy drink, absinthe, isn't it?! See, there's this great quote from him ... he says, "if your voices tell you not to paint, then paint, and the voices will be silenced". It's taking that control back. It's a fantastic statement.

### Recovery

For me, recovery is a very individual thing. I think it's been colonised in some ways. Sometimes I like the word "discovery". Because recovery says that I was ill. I wasn't ill. What I experienced was a consequence of my life experiences. So I thought "I've got to discover what happened in my life", and how do I alter that?

Recovery for me is having a quality of life that is acceptable to me. Where I can live and have control of my voices and my experiences. It's an individual thing, and I can function to a level that I want to function at.

I've heard a lot of people say, "we're always in recovery". I don't agree with that. I had my appendix out, I've recovered from it. I hear voices 24 hours a day, 7 days a week – yet I work 80-hour weeks now. I'm not always in recovery. As far as I'm concerned, I *am* recovered. It's a very individual thing. I think one thing you can't define recovery by is measured outcomes. It's not possible, because every human being is different.

Everyone has a different level to where they feel recovered.

### CHIME

I like that this is described as a framework. A framework is adaptable, it'll bend and bow to people's needs. A model is too rigid. You're trying to fit something into a box, and to me it becomes a square peg, round hole thing. If it doesn't work, as a system, we get a big mallet and we hammer them through. But when they come out the other side, you've still got the problems.

### Connectedness

Being connected with my children was a big one. I felt a little more privileged than a lot of people in psychiatric care. Because they didn't have children. And for me, they were a big focus. I wanted to stay connected with them. It was very hard at one time, to be really honest with you. Cause when I was with my first wife, and I went mad (that's my terminology), she threw me out of the family home. I was living on the streets for a while. She tried to keep me away from the children.

I don't take antipsychotics now, but at that time I was taking 25 drugs a day. I was walking like a robot. I'd have to get up at 6 o'clock in the morning, for what would be a 20-minute walk which used take me about 90 minutes. But I wanted my kids to know I was there, I wanted to be close to them. They were my driving force. And this is how crazy it might sound, but I wanted to be connected with them so much that I used to hide in the bushes outside the school. And as they walked past, Dad would pop out the bushes– "hi kids, how are you?". I always wanted to be there.

I think a massive thing in my recovery was when I stopped being as mad and I got a quality of life that was acceptable to me, all my children came to live with me. For me, that was so important. I had to keep moving on in with life, because I had a responsibility for three children.

*Hope*

I think hope is very important. As I always say, "depression never killed anyone. Hopelessness kills". I think I have been to that point myself. I have made attempts on my own life, but that's because I couldn't see a way out. And for me, that was because of the diagnosis that I was given. "Chronic schizophrenia". The psychiatrist actually said to me, "you'll never ever work again". Now I was used to being a bit of a workaholic – I'd had my own business turning a million pound a year over. Those words are so powerful. And this is why you have to try and develop hope. It's how the hopelessness can come in.

I had to create my own hope. And I got that, really, from attending a hearing voices group. I had many years on a psychiatric ward, and I never met anybody else with lived experience. They were there, but we weren't encouraged to talk about it. And when I went to a hearing voices group and I saw people had moved on in their lives, that created hope for me. That I can be where they are. Maybe not as far on, but I realised there was a way out. Without hope it's very difficult.

*Identity*

Well, that's a really good question isn't it! I can't actually sit here and tell you who I am. I can say "I'm Pete Bullimore, I've been married twice, I've got three children, I've got ten grandchildren." It doesn't actually tell you *who I am*, though. It tells you what I've done. And for a while, my identity became a chronic schizophrenic. That's who I was. That became my identity, because I didn't know who I was.

I went through a lot of childhood trauma. As a child (I didn't know this word back then), I used to dissociate. And one time I stayed out of my body too long. I don't know why I've come up with this number, Robert, but I think there's five percent of me missing. I don't actually know who I am as a whole person. I can say I've got an identity I'm happy with, but it's not the real me, because that's something that I lost in childhood that I can never find. So it's a difficult one that. But I was known as a chronic schizophrenic, and you see it so many times now. When we travel the world and go and visit Hearing Voices groups – "Hi my name's John, I'm paranoid schizophrenic"; "Hi my name's Mary, I'm bipolar" – your identity is formed by diagnosis. You lose the real self. That's how people introduce themselves.

Recovery can remove or replace an identity. In years gone I'd say, "I'm Pete, I'm a chronic schizophrenic", now I'd rather say, "I'm Pete, I'm a husband, I'm a father, I'm a grandfather". *That's* my identity – as a human being.

There is still a stigma there, though. If I'm working away from home I might go in a bar in the evening, and quite often people are nosey. "What you doing round here?". "I'm teaching on mental health, about hearing voices". "Why do you do that?". I'll say, "I'm a voice hearer". And they've got two options – they can talk to me about it, or they can walk away. But the majority of them, they'll stay and talk. I'm not ashamed to say I hear voices, and that's how I'm going to introduce myself. I am a voice hearer, and if you don't like it – it's your issue, not mine.

*Meaning*

My purpose is to help people not have to go through what I've been through. That's a big purpose for me. I'm not really interested in the money side of it. As I say, I had a business turning a million pound over a year, and that just brought me unhappiness. I'm driven to help others. I always say, if I won £10 million on the lottery, I would give it to people with mental health problems. I really would. If I can travel round the world (we delivered training in 13 different countries in 2019), talk about my experiences, and change one person's life, give them hope to change and create an identity who they want to be, then all of those 8 years of abuse that I went through has been worth it. I think for me, that's really important.

I'm a wounded healer, and everybody in our organisation says the same. I think it's quite widespread that. If we can stop other people going through the difficult things we went through, then everything's worth it.

*Empowerment*

For me, I sit here, and I have to say that I have been lucky. Because of the people that I've met in life … I met a guy, a psychologist from Manchester who was inspirational in the Hearing Voices movement, Terry McLoughlin. I was the archetypical schizophrenic, and he took me under his wing. People I'm going to mention, some of them you might have heard of – an Emeritus professor of psychiatry called Alec Jenner, he was known around the world. And Terry introduced me to him. It was a great education, a wealth of knowledge. Then people like Professor John Reid, Professor Richard Bentall, Professor Marius Romme, Professor Bob Johnson, all these people you would never meet at just one university. But they're all personal friends, and they accepted me for who I was.

For me, that became empowering. Famous professionals letting me have a conversation and listening to what I tell them. Not saying "we're the professionals, you're not". That acceptance of being brought into their lives. You can have the divide, "you're just a voice hearer, we're the academics". But it was so empowering that these people accepted me for being Pete, not for being a chronic schizophrenic.

Like with Marius Romme, he's the professor who started the Hearing Voices movement. I've known him for about 30 years now. It might seem nothing, but when I got married to Linda in 2014, he came to our wedding. That's empowering – somebody so famous coming to a voice hearer's wedding. Little things like that. Being recognised for the changes you're trying to make by such important people, that's empowering. Him talking to me as a friend, not as a patient.

## Creativity

Creativity for me, it's making the best of things that you can and finding a different way out of it. You've got to be creative to survive. Especially around voice hearing, it's really understanding it from a metaphorical perspective. I have three external voices and two internal voices, they're my main voices. And in some ways, they're all creative. The external voices are there 24/7, even now. They continually call me a murderer. "Murderer, murderer, murderer". It used to be horrible to hear – it's still horrible to hear now, but I understand it better. Basically, my voices are a part of me. They're not a separate entity. They are linked to my emotions.

When I was 23, I had a son who died. There's nothing that I could have done to save him, but it's guilt. That's when they started to call me a murderer. It wasn't until later in life when I thought "my voices are a part of me, it's my emotions, what do I need to address here?". Basically, what they're saying is "unless you deal with the guilt, you'll always feel like a murderer". So that's the creative part of me.

Another voice I know is my creative side, which got crushed in childhood. When I was four, I could write. Not a lot, but I used to write short stories for the teachers at nursery and they always liked them. When the abuse started, I felt it got crushed.

When my mum died (I was 34), I got this voice that just said, "a village called Pumpkin". I thought "what's that?". But it wouldn't answer any questions. It would just keep giving me all these silly names of people, I had this urge to write them down. And then it said, "a children's book". I thought "I'm not reading a children's book!" The voice said, "write it". I thought "I can't write children's books". But then it gave me a theme and the chapter just flowed. It took me three years to write it, but when the book got published that voice disappeared. And the book was sold all over the world, it's been fantastic. Now I've started to write another children's book with my grandchildren, and I don't need that voice because my creative side has come back.

To me, that voice embodied my creativity. What confused me was it sounds like a female. It's not my voice, it's a female voice. But it is my creative side. What I was told by someone, and I looked this up and I know it's correct, whether it's musicians, authors, poets, we all have a creative side. And often 90% of them who hear a voice they will hear it as a female voice. But it is part of you. So, I know that's my creative side now.

## Creativity being crushed

That had a really devastating impact, to be honest. I had three abusers. It was a female the first one. When she started to hurt me, and I mean really hurt me, that's when I stopped being creative. I kind of shut down. Then she brought another female in to be involved, and I developed these feelings of self-loathing. And then she brought a male figure to be involved, and it went on for 8 years. And that self-loathing became a very deep self-hatred. I hated Peter (myself). I did not want to be him, and I could never find anything nice about him.

When my dad died (I didn't expect it, he had a massive heart attack), I looked at my life and I thought "why do I hate myself so much? I never do anything for myself, I always do for others". And I managed to let some of this self-hatred go, and that's when that voice came. I think because I'd let some of that hatred go, that was my creative side coming back. It's been locked away by all those negative feelings.

### Creativity and recovery

Creativity definitely helped with my recovery, because I look at things differently now. I can be more creative with the voices. When they say negative things, I can work it out from a creative perspective. These voices are a part of you – what's the real message they're trying to tell you? I find that really, really helpful.

Even when I'm working, I do a lot of one-to-one work with people, and I present case studies on training. People say "how did you think of that? I would never have thought to say that to that person". It just comes into my mind – I walk away and I reflect, "What is the real message here?". And it takes me a bit of time to work it out, but 9 times out of 10 it is fairly accurate when I go back to them. It's like solving a puzzle, very much so.

### Creativity and voice hearing

I always give an example, talking about the metaphors – you've got a 14-year-old boy, developing his sexuality, he's going through puberty. He gets sexually abused by a woman. How's his body going to respond? There is going to be arousal, there's nothing he can do about it as sexual organs are governed by the brain. But the abuser will tell him it's his fault. "If you don't get aroused, I can't have sex with you". They'll blame you. All these things that they say.

Now if we don't deal with that, and it manifests into voices. Those voices won't say "get some therapy for your trauma, will you mate?". No! They'll constantly repeat what the abusers said. Now, what these voices are doing, they're being very supportive. They're talking about things in your life you have not dealt with. So, you talk about voices being messengers that bring awful messages, but don't shoot the messenger. If you look at what the real meaning is behind it, then you can understand what the voices are telling you to do. When you deal with that under-pinning problem, it takes the power away from the voices.

You'll never understand a person's experience without a comprehensive narrative. Narratives are important. When services say, "don't listen to voices", it's absolute nonsense. You've got to listen to voices. If you've got a four-year-old girl, you're cooking dinner, if she wants your attention she'll get it. "Dad" – "Just a minute" – "Dad!" – "Just a minute" – she'll keep shouting! And that's what a voice will do. "I'm going to shout at you until you listen to me. I'm trying to tell you something here, I'm trying to help you". We have to look at it from the metaphorical perspective, it's important.

Voices are messages, the voices are trying to be creative. They're not going to give it to you easy! This is your creativity for yourself, trying to make sense of this. And that's why when we give people heavy medication, it blocks their cognitions. You can't think creatively to make sense of it. That's one of the problems. Understanding the voices, that is empowering.

So it has definitely played a big role in my recovery, creativity. I couldn't do what you're doing, Robert. I couldn't go to university to learn, I don't have the attention span. I'm an experiential learner. When people say something, I can put it across from a different perspective. I'm not an academic, but I think in different ways to other people, and I explain things in different ways. Sometimes it's simpler to be more practical in your thinking. I think sometimes what I did really find helpful was drawing as well. I'm not a very good artist, but I always enjoyed it, because sometimes I couldn't verbalise what I was thinking and trying to say. But drawing it, and then having an art therapist ask, "what do you mean by this, Peter?", then I could explain it differently. That creative side was really important.

### Creativity in therapy

Painting was a creative way for me to get out what I was trying to say. Some of these drawings were very childlike, but that was the child that was still in me, explaining what had happened. We've all got that inner child. We have to change our thinking and see things through an adult's eyes not a child's eyes and it helps us grow into an adult emotionally, but at times I've felt like the five-year-old boy that was getting hurt.

That's why my paintings came out how they did. And then the art therapist would say – "So, how old do you think you were, Pete, when this happened?". I said, "I was five". And I didn't speak like a child, but I felt like that child. But when we could work through them, I started to grow emotionally. Because I was heard, I was believed. But I could never have verbally told her, or anyone.

It's like a different language to express things in. Because, quite often what happens when you've been through childhood trauma, you can regress to the age when it happened. It's called "Infantilism". Now when I went back to feeling like a five-year-old boy, I didn't have adult vocabulary. I didn't know the words that I needed, but by drawing it, then she could say to me "is this what you're telling me?". And then I could say "yes".

So that for me was really important. I did a painting, and it got put in an art exhibition. I've actually still got it. But it was Anne the art therapist who said "Pete, can you paint yourself?". And this is how I saw myself in the mirror; I was on all fours, crouched over, my body was yellow. Half my face was red, half my face was brown, with a big split down the middle.

I said, "that's me, that's what I was looking at as I painted it". And she said, "I'm trying to make sense of this Pete, what you trying to tell me?". I said, "that's me, it's what I see in the mirror" – "So what is it you're actually seeing?" – "I don't know who I am any more. I'm so disjointed. I don't know who Pete is, I don't see him anymore, he's gone". That's how I could express how I felt. I don't exist anymore, because I'd been written off in society, by the system. What's the point in looking like a human being anymore? But if I walk down the street looking like that, people will see me. I'm not invisible anymore. I'd become invisible, nobody was interested in me apart from when they were giving me antipsychotics. It had stripped me of my identity, a chronic schizophrenic is all that I am now. But through doing the painting, I became a person again. It did really well in this exhibition, when I explained to people what it meant.

Once I was stood just looking at the painting at the exhibition. This man and woman came in who obviously didn't know who I was. They were looking at the painting, and he said to her "he must be so unwell whoever has that's painted that". I didn't say anything, I thought "actually I'm not unwell. I'm trying to create my identity. It's a statement from me, and you're misreading the whole thing". I'm wondering why he doesn't think "what is this person trying to tell us?". It's so easy to say, "he's unwell". If I'm unwell, then it doesn't matter what my abusers did to me. It's because I've got an illness. Whereas I'm trying to tell a story here. How did I come to see myself in this way? And people have got to be creative when they ask people about their experiences. Because there's a message in there. We can't always verbalise, but there's a way to do things to find out what the story is. Without creativity, I'd find it hard to be here today.

### Changing meanings in creative works

As I wrote my book, I didn't pick up on a lot of the things that were in there. And as I say, it sold all over the world, even the Royal Library in Denmark bought a copy! It probably is sold more to professionals than children to be honest. But I've had so many calls from psychiatrists and psychologists that I know – "I've read your book, Pete. Lots of your life in there." I say "where?". But when you point it out … Like when I was a little boy, I used to go and hide in the woods instead of going to school, cause I felt intimidated by some of the teachers. One of the stories is about the guy who spent time in the woods, and he saw figures in trees and faces and all things like that. And I'd never noticed that. So for me, that was me telling my life in a different way. And probably in a way that I couldn't express some of the things that I didn't know as I was doing it.

Some people have picked up on this, I'd not looked at it any deeper. Because I didn't feel heard as a child. I tried to do everything that I could to raise awareness that I was being hurt, but my parents missed it – I don't blame them. Sometimes I didn't feel heard in services. I was saying "you're giving me all of these drugs, and I'm really struggling. I'm tired, I've dyskinesia, I'm in a hell of a state." And this one story, I can laugh about it now … there's a flock of sheep, and they're orange. It's the orange lambs of Pump Lane. The mum gets injured, and I think "oh I don't really want to let the mother sheep die". But then I had to bring a vet in, and I hadn't got a vet in the chapter. And I'm writing this on a Sunday morning,

Linda's sat across the other side of the room, and I said to this vet … right, vet has to save the sheep.

And you know in films if you get a line then you get more money? I heard this vet say to me "what line am I going to say?". I said "you're not saying anything. Save the sheep." – "No, I want a line" – "Look, will you save the sheep?" – "No, not unless I get a line"- "Will you save the bloody sheep?". And Linda said, "who you talking to?" – "This bloody vet won't save the sheep". So I had to write him a line so he would save the sheep … but actually, he wants to be heard. I was silenced, and I was silencing him. So, when I looked at it, actually there is a lot of me in there. He's allowed to be heard, why not? If I silence him, I've become part of the system that shuts people down.

### Creative inspiration and motivation

When the voice gave me a theme, they wouldn't repeat it. I had to get it there and then! We were travelling on a plane, and this voice came and gave the me the theme to a chapter – I had to get a vomit bag and write it down on that so I wouldn't forget it!

I've finished another book that's just being proofread at the moment. It's called *Making Sense of Paranoia*, and it's taken me 15 years to write it to be really honest with you. Since we've been in lockdown, I thought I need to be doing something. And it really opened my mind again, because we've done it a little bit differently. Now if you look at books, they usually start with a theory, then put the personal experiences at the end. And I thought "I'm going to turn this on its head – let's start with the narratives". We're looking at narratives of people who have been in services, and looking at some narratives of people who are paranoid but have never been in services. Some of them are very powerful. We're going to put the theory at the end. Does the theory fit the life experience, not the other way around. Because you can't have theory without the lived experience. So, I was thinking about it in a totally different way, thanks to that space from not travelling all the time with work. I've not enjoyed the lockdown, but it's helped me get that book finished!

### Creative process

I'm a creative thinker in a lot of things to be honest with you. I think a lot of people think the ideas I come up with are quite weird, quite bizarre. But I think I look at things in a more creative way. People think life's black and white – it isn't.

You've got to look holistically, look at the bigger picture. I teach a lot of psychiatrists, and they walk into this trap every time. I just say, "you're behaviour obsessed" – "Behaviour is primary, Pete" – "No it's not".

I say, "I can walk you all into a trap. Imagine you're in a relationship if you aren't already. You go home from work this evening, you walk through your front door, whoever you live with comes out the front room, punch you in the nose, run upstairs and slam the bedroom door. What do you do?" Inevitably, they reply "follow them upstairs!" – "Then what?", I ask. "To demand an explanation!" – "Exactly, thank you very much – you've walked straight into the trap. Why have they hit me? Why are people behaving in a certain way? What has created the anger?"

It's like with people with mental health problems – they'll behave in certain ways, because they're trying to tell you something! "I'm angry cause you're not listening to me!". And so you've got to be creative, you've got to think beyond that. Like my eldest daughter, she's quite senior in a mental health trust now. She was on the ward the other week, and this guy was an ex-boxer. He's run down the ward and punched her straight in the face. So they've got him, put him in seclusion as you can imagine. "Right, we're going to move him to forensic". And she said "no, you're not. He's going nowhere" – "But, he's attacked you." – "No no no. He's angry with someone, and whoever he's angry with, they're not here. If he goes to forensic, no one is going to ask him. He's staying here, and I'm going to find out who he really wanted to hit". My daughter thinks very much like me. Find out why he's done it, or you're never going to solve the problem. You've got to think creatively about things.

It's looking at narratives, people's stores. That is a way of helping people to heal.

### Artisticness versus creativity

I don't think there is a difference to be honest. I think you've got to be creative to do art, haven't you? I think it's a side that's in some people. I think we can *all* be creative. I think we can *all* be artistic, though there's probably different levels of how the art will look. Some are really excellent artists. For me, it's more about what the story is behind it. Every picture tells a story. And I think that's the most important thing.

I think anything can be art, really. Like you get a lot of graffiti now, don't you? And some of them are very talented artists, Banksy and people like that. Some of it is just like a scrawl, but what does it mean to them? It means something to someone. What is it – someone trying to be seen? Trying to be heard?

There's someone round here, I don't know who it is, keeps writing "Dyson" all over. And I think, is that something to do with the hoover factory, something like that? But he's even wrote it on the back of the toilet door, now. There's something in that. It doesn't *look* artistic, but when you look at it again, it's all very symmetrical. How's he doing it? Some of it's sprayed, some is written. There are never any flaws in it. So I'm wondering … there's something behind that. In its own way, there is artistic creativity in there. There's a mystery behind it, and it makes you think. Is that not what art is meant to do?

### How the creativity of others helps

It helps in different ways. I've always liked the work of Van Gogh. I knew he was a voice hearer, and I know there was a story behind all the pictures. But I think from another context as well, with people I've met, like I said with Bob Johnson and Terry and people like that. They thought creatively, away from the medical model.

That was a big influence on me. Looking at it differently. I'm not this flawed human being. This is a perfectly normal reaction to the things that have happened in my life. It's not an illness … it's *made* me ill. But it's not an illness.

And I think seeing the world differently, having different perspectives about myself made a massive difference. I realised then … antipsychotics can't cure anything, there's nothing to cure. So I *need* to be off them. Otherwise I can't do anything, my thinking was blocked. I couldn't think clearly. I didn't even know what day it was. So I needed to be off them so I could think clearly and understand the world and the perspective around me again. I wouldn't have had that creativity if I had stayed on all those drugs, and that creativity allowed me to start processing what had happened to me.

I could see patterns and associations again. I went to a workshop in Sheffield where a lady talked about her life, and how she was abused as a child. And "what had happened to me as a child went on for so long, in some ways I knew it was wrong. But it just became part of me". And when I heard her talk about it … *boof*.

All these memories came back. I could see the associations. Sometimes it's just hearing someone else say it. And I remember getting in the bath, and I'm laid at home thinking "why have I not seen this before?". I think it's just because I'd been indoctrinated with "it's an illness. You've got chronic schizophrenia. You must take these drugs. There's something wrong with your brain". Nobody scanned my brain. Not one person! So how do you know it's anything wrong with it then?! I was just making these associations and thinking … I need to be off these drugs. And then I could see it totally differently.

It was a similar thing seeing Van Gogh's art. Everybody says it was through the absinthe. It wasn't. Van Gogh was a voice hearer as well, and he actually talked about how the voices helped him do some of these paintings. They helped him be creative. I always liked Van Gogh's sunflowers. I've actually got that on the wall. It's not his, it's mine! I did it in art therapy with pastels, but I did it just with my finger, nothing else.

It's one of the best ones I've ever done. It's hung up in the flat. I like it to be where it is, because every time I see it, it shows me how far I've come. When I did that I was, in my words, mad. I was off my head. But I managed to do it, and I think "I am not going back there. Not for anyone." So it's a bit of a driving force, as well.

You've got to keep one step ahead, that's the important thing. We all have days – I'm only human. But then … I'm very fortunate, I've got a very supportive partner, Linda. And sometimes, certain times like April and May (both my parents died in April, my son died in May), the voices get quite difficult, and I can be up in the night, wandering around thinking. Linda will ask what is wrong I say, "I can't work this out and what's going on in my mind", and she will say "you're trying too hard". Linda will ask "if one of your clients was saying this to you, what advice would you give them?". And then when I'm not focusing on me, I'm thinking about someone else, I'll come up with an answer, and she'll say "well, why don't you take your own advice?". Sometimes you just need that support to be thinking a different way as well.

### Creativity museum metaphor

I tell you, I kept that picture which showed how I describe myself, I've still got the sunflowers, but I actually threw all the others away. Linda wasn't very happy that I'd done that, but what it was ... I cleaned all the office out, and I saw them, and ... the reason I threw them away is that I was a bit disappointed in myself. I thought "how did I let myself get that low?". I always thought I was one step ahead of everybody else. But mental health doesn't come with a calling card. Before you know it, bang. It's got you. And it's easy to reflect and say I should have seen this, I should have seen that. But I didn't ... To be honest with you, Robert, I was disgusted with myself. That I'd let myself get that low, living on the streets, things like that. I thought, I *need* to get rid of these pictures. It's my past, it's gone. Some memories I don't want to be reminded of. I took charge of the story I was telling with the pictures, and kept the ones that still spoke to me.

### Creativity as a risk

Sometimes you can think a bit *too* far outside the box! Can be a little bit *too* creative, like. I sometimes do think too deeply into things, maybe looking for something that's not there. It's helpful when people point it out to you – it's usually my kids that do that!

### Everyday creativity

I really like cooking. It's a great retreat for me. Respite. I do a lot of cooking on a Saturday. I'm working 80 hours a week, and I'm shattered at the end of it. But I can go in the kitchen, and I like baking. I like making pasties, pies, cake, things like that. Linda leaves me in there, and I can be there for 6 hours. I cook, and I listen to the music, I have a glass of wine.

But where the creativity comes in even more is – I won't waste anything. I may have got a little bit of pastry left ... I'm not throwing that away. I've got to cook something with this! So, I get creative. For example, I looked in the cupboard and I found a bag of chocolate raisins. I'm going to make a chocolate raisin pie. I put the chocolate raisins in, screwed it up, egg washed it and put it in the cooker and cooked it. I said to Linda, "What do you think to this?" She said, "That's fantastic!" I have to be creative, what can I cook differently?

And even daft as it sounds – washing the floors. I wash all the floors in the apartment. But I think "hold on, is there a better way of doing this? So I don't have to keep moving that? And I can't do it this way, cause if I walk in there, that floors still going to be wet. I've got to think a different way around this". So, everything I do, I have to try and be creative and get the best out of it.

In some ways it's about control. I've always got to have control in my life. I never want to control another human being, but I've *must* have control in *my* life. I know what it's like *not* to have that control.

Now this is going to sound really barmy what I'm going to say now, but when I go shopping with Linda, we have a shopping trolley. And I always pack the shopping trolley, 'cause I always say it should be a competition – the Best Shopping Trolley Packer in the World! And I'm going to win it! So I'll be there "that's got to go in first, put the bottle in next". I always find a creative way so that we don't have to have a carrier bag as well as the trolley. I'll get everything in! Maybe we could be rivals in the competition, Robert!

| | |
|---|---|
| *Robert:* | I am grateful to Peter for so clearly demonstrating creativity as a therapeutic tool – in art therapy, and with his voices. A key theme through our conversation was the use of creative thinking in understanding others – that practitioners must try to think flexibly and with creativity when working with people facing mental health difficulties. An important message. It shows how creativity is a tool by which we can communicate, and that works both ways. |

## References

Cordle, H., Fradgley, J., Carson, J., Holloway, F., & Richards, P. (Eds.) (2011). *Psychosis: Stories of recovery and hope*. Quay Books.

PowAnimate. (2014). Peter Bullimore – The power of the narrative [video]. www.youtube.com/watch?v=5DBXm0eanjA.

# 9    StoryTeller – ANON

*ANON and Robert Hurst*

> *Robert:*   This chapter is a little different. The author has decided to remain anonymous. ANON was the only participant in the research that was recruited via my connections. We knew of each other via a friend of a friend, and had chatted in the few instances where we met. ANON had always very openly spoken about her difficulties with mental health, her "crumbles" as she refers to them. I also knew of ANON as a highly creative person. She is one of those people whose creativity you can sense when you meet them. It pours from her even in a casual conversation.
>
> By trade, she is an actor and a writer. Specifically, she works with comedy. It shows. My biggest hope for ANON's chapter is that I am able to capture the hilarity that she radiates. Whether it is with fun accents or razor-sharp comments, ANON is always on the ball, making people smile and laugh. That is what I knew going into this. When ANON agreed to be involved, I was delighted. I hope you can see why.

## ANON's story

My dad died when I was really young, quite suddenly. Bit intense that, isn't it? But I suppose it is the best place to start to explain my head. There's a lot of traumas with it. I shouldn't laugh … I'm not laughing at *that*. But it's funny, because the stuff I write always has death in it. I don't know why …

Well, I do …

### Recovery

Recovery to me means learning to navigate your normality. I feel there's too many times where you're told that you're *going* to be fixed, or that you *have* to be fixed. And there comes a point where you realise it's just you, and you just need to figure

DOI: 10.4324/9781003319405-9

out your own path. You just get to a point where you stop hating yourself. That would be my view of recovery – learning to see the ups with it, trying to stop seeing it as such a negative hold … it's got positive attributes as well.

I don't see it as trying to be "cured". How morbid can we get? I think I told someone once not to try and fix me, 'cause I will die as someone who has got all these conditions. I just want to not be at 11 out of 10. I'll settle for 7. Just let me get by!

What I realised is that it's just about navigating it. I was having a massive relapse, in my early twenties. There was an issue at work where colleagues were mocking me for my mental health, and I just stopped. My head was just … sick of it. Sick of being mocked, of being treated a different way by people who haven't experienced these things, who don't understand it. I think that's what it took for me. It just clicked. People can mock you for having it, but I'm glad they've never had to live with what I have. Then I stopped seeing everything as negative, and instead of seeing myself as broken, I thought … I am just me. And I'm not gonna let other people try and make me think that I'm ill when I'm just … me!

### CHIME

*Connectedness*

I won't lie, if I've "crumbled" (this is what I call my mental health relapses) and I've got really bad, I'm well-known for going off-grid. I don't want people knowing that it's got hold of me again. It used to be out of guilt, when I was younger. Of feeling like I've failed. I grew up in quite an intense household, where you couldn't be weak or fail. So I always used to hide it if I was really struggling.

However, the older I've gotten, especially in the last few years, it's more a case that going off-grid is beneficial for me. It is taking time for me. It's selfish in a good way – I can just say no and not talk to people while I get my head straight. And if people don't respect it, they don't. But I think recovery-wise, connectedness … I'm very bad for it. I will either cut people off, or I will go to meet up with people but then just get too anxious and bail. I think I'll always be a little hermit!

*Hope*

The older I've got, the more it is possible for me to not laugh at you talking about "hope". If you'd met early-twenties ANON and asked about that, you'd have prob-ably got a big swear word said back to you. But now I'm about to turn 30, I think I have more hope that I will get a lot better, not even recovery-wise. I'll still have crumbles, and I'm ok with that now. I won't hate myself for it. I have hope that I will stop being as cruel to myself when I do have them. Instead, I'll let myself have it and think "you've got through it again". Because I have hope for being more kind to myself.

*Identity*

When I hit 25, I didn't care if people identified me with mental health. It didn't bother me anymore. Whereas in my early twenties as I started being diagnosed with a few more things, I was very angry to be told "you have this, you have that". I very much felt like I was just getting pigeon-holed, and I didn't want to be. So I was very… angry. But now I'm older, I am open about my mental health. It doesn't faze me, I'm quite proud to have got to the age that I've got. Which makes me sounds like I'm 60 but I know I'm not. But to have gotten to the age I've got to with everything that I've gone through, and the mental health that I've got, and still not be ashamed of it anymore… I don't care anymore, it's me!

*Meaning*

Recovery and meaning… I'm definitely not there yet! I think that's one of the things that I really struggle with. I put a lot of pressure on myself. I have all my social media on timers, cause my head can just get so bad – everyone does with social media – but especially if I see someone else succeeding. For some reason instead of just being like "wow, you've done great", my head will punish me. "Why isn't that you?". So I'm probably not too great with that one.

　　Though, I suppose I find meaning in sharing my experiences to help others. That's a nice way to think about it, actually. When I was younger I used to hate everything that ever happened to me, and how my head was. Then the older I get, there's part of me thinking I can help people who are going through aspects of it, which is something I never got before. So I suppose yeah, I find some meaning there.

*Empowerment*

At the moment, I think I feel very empowered about my mental health. I'm very maternal with anyone who seems to be having a bit of mental health difficulty. I don't want anyone to feel as isolated and persecuted as I was made to. Going through my teenage years, getting diagnosed in my early twenties … it still wasn't accepted back then. I was made to feel that I was a hypochondriac in school. So now in my late twenties, I want to give people the safe space that I didn't have. I feel that is a massive empowerment thing for me. I'm very empowered to have mental health difficulties, I see it as good and bad. But one day I'm gonna be more good than bad with it … One day.

**Creativity**

Creativity means to me … to play. It's so weird, it's like I'm a paradox of myself – my mental health tries to restrict my head, very much, but the creative side of me wants to play. Wants to live in the moment … The main thing with my creativity is just to try and enjoy life more. Which is the polar opposite of the depressive part of my head.

Robin Williams said something along the lines of "the saddest people are normally the happiest, and try to make people the happiest because they don't want them to feel how they felt". I think that's probably a massive tick in the box for me as to why I do character comedy, stand-up and clowning. I have very self-deprecating, defensive humour, which sadly I got as a child. But I always want to make people feel happy, and make sure everyone is comfortable. I think that is the part of me trying to protect the young me that never had it. The creativity works as a kind of defence.

Because I'm actually quite shy. When I'm off-stage, it's like I can breathe a bit more and be quiet. I get very socially anxious; I get really stressed in big crowds. But people never believe it, because I'll go and do big character comedy in massive wigs, and mess about. But it's just a different mask that I can put on. I do think it's a protection thing, just to be stupid.

So I do think creativity for me it just lets me be a bit more free. It lets me enjoy life, not to get stuck in what people tell me I've got to do. With creativity I can just do whatever my brain wants to do. And people that have seen my work, they will see that I do whatever my head thinks of … and I shouldn't be allowed to a lot of the time!

### Creativity as work

But then you've got the awful, horrible side of creativity where you get consumed with ego and jealousy and trying to be the best you can be. God what am I doing in this profession? It's not healthy, is it? You always feel … inferior. You're picked up on for how you sound, how you look. I've had so many comments about my appearance, that I have developed a hatred for how I look. I cannot stand it. That's because of the profession I'm in. People think that they can do that. And you get told a lot in the business that you have to have a thick skin to do it. I hate that. I don't think you should have to have a thick skin to do anything. I just think people shouldn't be arseholes.

Acting-wise, the amount of my friends that definitely have undiagnosed mental health issues… . You're so anxious, you feel like you've gotta constantly be putting yourself out there or you'll get forgotten about. And so sometimes you just burn out … I'm really bad for burning out.

I used to do videos every week – comedy videos. And I just couldn't cope with it. There was so much pressure to do it that my creativity stopped. My head was so overwhelmed with checking how many people had liked it, comparing the stats to other videos. Thinking that means people must hate me. My depression just came along and claimed everything. So compared to many of my acting mates, I have a lot more restrictions.

When you interact with other people from the profession, you're taught that it's "networking". You should be trying to get something from it. I've always died socially, so I never met anybody. I was really bad at it! "Hello, goodbye!"

But actors don't ask how you are. When they meet each other they ask, "what have you been up to?". And no matter what the intent of the question was, your actor head will automatically assume they want to know what acting work you've done, and you start to list it and it's just not healthy. I think Heath Ledger even said once that actors "don't talk to each other as humans, it's always about competition and survival of the fittest". So now I always make sure I ask, "how are you?", and if they start to tell me about acting I say, "No, no, no, I don't care … How are *you*?".

I'd rather try and breathe and enjoy being creative and get through life than try and spin every plate and not cope. I've done that, and it's not worth it. It really isn't.

### Actively pursuing success

The thing with success is how you view it. So for some people to be successful, they can be doing freelance work. Just enough to get by, but they still have their foot in the door. For some people they have to be on TV. For example, you'll have actors who have worked for years, and they'll get a small role on TV, and it'll say "newcomer". No. They've been grafting for years and years.

It's very competitive. I've got something written on my little board here that says, "someone else's success is not your failure". There's this girl who is a different casting to me, but the same age. We both do comedy. We're mates, so when one of us is doing well we're happy, but then we're also consumed with complete jealousy and worry about the other taking your spot. I think as women we're taught that there's not many spaces for us in the profession, so it's even more competitive. She looks nothing like me. I'm the height of a child, she's not. She's from down south, I'm not. There's no way we would ever compete for the same job. But society has made us think there can only be one funny woman that we know. And we would literally hate each other, but be mates still, but also die when the other was doing well. Whereas now, we actually try and breathe. We will openly say to each other – "I'm struggling".

That competitiveness is really bad for creativity. Sometimes you want to make something just to beat someone, which is pathetic. You're not doing creativity to be creative, it's your mental health grasping you – "You're missing your chance, you need to do this, you're not good enough". Sometimes you just make something for the sake of having something out there. To do one better. When you're in that cycle, you're never going to make good work, because you're not doing it for the right reasons. You're consumed with everything else.

### Creative process

I always have notebooks with me. No matter what bag I've got, it has to fit a notebook in, and I'll vomit-write things. I'm naughty for this at work … I'll always be writing little things down.

My main thing is listening to music. Music has saved me so many times. If anything is really bad, I just block it out by putting my headphones on. I put music on, then my brain goes into its carefree world, and I start to come up with random ideas. The last play I wrote started with me writing a stupid song for my own entertainment. It entertained my boyfriend and my best mate, and they encouraged me to carry on. That ended up becoming a play. Same with the one I'm writing now.

I'll just sit down and just have a random idea in my brain – I can see it, and how I want it to look. And I'll normally giggle to myself and look like an absolute weirdo. Then I'll start typing it up and keep coming back to it. I've got something called "The Bible", and it's got all of my stuff in that hasn't become "something" yet. So I can always nick things and move bits around.

### Impact of mental health on creativity

If my mental health has too much of a hold on me, I can't be creative. My head just won't picture things or do things, and then I get wound up at it. Whereas when I feel like I can breathe, then I will be able to just be quite happy with my thoughts, jot things down.

If my depression gets me, and I have to be creative, I can't do anything. I waste so much time where I could be doing something by beating myself up that I'm not doing anything, and looking at everyone else doing something. I go in that vicious hypothetical horrendous cycle.

And I get these thoughts – "You're failing, what are you doing with your life, look at your age, what are you doing". All my mates have their own houses and everything like that. And even though they're still jealous of me for doing freelance stuff, if my head's bad, I just look at them and think "what the fuck, ANON? What are you doing wearing wigs?"

### Impact of creativity on mental health

Creativity has helped with my recovery because I think it has let me vocalise things that I didn't know how to process. I've had quite a few traumas. Having those locked inside you is not healthy. So I think creativity-wise, I might let it out through writing. I have quite dark humour, so I might have a little joke about it. And it's empowering – where other people might say you shouldn't joke about stuff like that, for me it's a little bit of freedom. A little nod to say that I *can* speak about it. I think it helped me get through so much, developing creativity and humour. To learn how to cope in the world, cause otherwise I just had to "get on with everything", and I didn't know how. So, I went to the Muppets, 'cause I was only really young. Things like that, where it was so daft, and it just seemed so fun and … It wasn't my life.

I think that really made me want to be creative with funny things. If it wasn't for being creative and messing about and making things that make me laugh, joking about things that might have happened to me – I think I would be in a much worse place. I don't think my recovery would be what it is. I don't think I'd be as empowered as I am with mental health. I think I would have been lost to the stigma and horrendously unhappy – this is coming from a depressive! Whereas I think creativity has allowed me, when I was ready, to succeed with it. To not view myself as being broken.

### Creativity as way of reframing/processing

It's quite morbid, but there will always be some nod to death in my work. A joke about someone not understanding that something is dead, be it a joke animal or something. Everyone else will laugh at it, and I'll be laughing, but I know the undercurrent of it is my childhood trauma. Being able to openly say "this is how I cope". Come to my little crazy world where I'm gonna mess about in wigs, and I'm gonna make jokes about death, and you're all gonna laugh and you're gonna go home and be like "what a funny scene". But in reality, that's six-year-old me asking "how do I cope?" This is the way.

So I do think it's helped me to recover, to learn how to carry on. Because you can't just stop. Nothing is gonna change what happened to you. So you just have to navigate, and you will crumble. That's why I like "navigate". Because when you first go into CBT, you're given this illusion that you're going to get fixed. It won't bother you anymore. And then a few months down the line, you're the same. So what I do is take negative things, and try to make them positive. I joke about it. The creative side of my jokey head says, "let's make up a silly story".

If I'm completely honest there's still a lot of stuff that I haven't healed from. There's a lot that I won't touch. My humour is completely defensive, it's my protection. I feel like I joke about it because I don't want to really think about it, because if I think too much about it, it's very sad. When I've openly told people about it, they get very sad, and they say, "you've had a very sad life", and … yeah. But I've never known a different one. That's just the life that I have had.

Creativity allowed me to not wallow quite as much when I could breathe. I had a lot of bad years with depression, but creativity allowed me to see the fun again. Joke around again. It allowed me to make comments on crap things that had happened, and even if no one understands that I've made a joke about something being dead because of my underlying traumas, it's a little sigh of relief for me. I got that little bit of poison out again.

There's another dead thing in this play I'm writing, actually! When I read it to my best mate, she just said, "oh for God's sake!" and I just think it's going to be in everything that I do. There's always some joke about death. It's my calling card!

### Consuming the creativity of others

For me, one hundred per cent. A thousand per cent! I had to escape the world I was in, and I went to *Muppet Treasure Island*. I went to Mel Brooks. All the daft slapstick comedies where there wasn't an undertone to it, really. In the Muppets there is, but it's so daft that you can just forget everything that's going on in your life and be happy.

That's what I do with my writing, there's no underlying thing. I normally do historical stuff, cause I'm a history nerd. I put little bits of history for you to learn, maybe get you interested. But my goal when I write stuff is to create something that makes me laugh, and hope that it makes others laugh too. And that's it. I don't want to make you think about your sad lives, I don't want you to think about socio-economic stuff that we're all stuck in. Maybe I'll hint at it, but my main goal is to make people laugh.

As an actor, I sometimes get slated because I don't go to the theatre much. My view is, why do I want to go watch something that's going to make me sad? My life is already sad. I will go and watch a clown show, a comedy show – something where the goal is just to make you laugh. I suppose that's a link for recovery as well, without realising it! Everything I create, the only goal is just to make you laugh. To make you forget about everything that has happened. I think that's what links it to my childhood – to be creative helped me forget everything that had happened. So now that I'm an adult, my goal is to do that for other people.

You've had a rubbish day? Watch me in a wig!

Something bad is happening? Watch this really weird play!

When I did my play people called it "wonderfully weird". "It's really cheered me up, it's so strange". That's all I wanted. I just wanted people to breathe. I don't feel like you can ever breathe anymore. My creativity and my work is pure escapism.

### Creating for success – art versus creativity

I think some people make stuff just for their egos. We're all guilty of it, I've made stuff to make myself look good, and then hated it because it's not me. It's not my ethos. And I just look at it like "you absolute bell end, why?!". But you do it! Because you get caught up in the pressure of the industry and society. If I can be creative and it is the way I want it to be, it will always be to create art. It will always to be, for me, something for people to escape in. To have a laugh with. Nothing else, just go have fun.

Sadly, I don't think some people do it that way. Some people create stuff just to get the extra praise, or just to be seen. I don't think that art is always creative. As humans we are all flawed, and I don't think everyone will admit that. I happily admit that I've got flaws, which is why I think I'm more at peace with myself. I don't think other people will admit that they've got egos, and they do things a certain way. I fully admit it. I have an ego. I'm an actor, how could I lie? I will do things for praise, yes. But if that's my sole intention, it won't be good, and I won't be happy with it.

Aiming only for success with creativity is going about it the wrong way. It won't be your best work, I promise you. With any artist. When you put the pressure on yourself to write something just to achieve, it's not gonna be the best work and you won't achieve anything. Whereas if you just write something just to write, to release your soul a bit, to do what you need to do to be you – it'll be amazing.

During lockdown, for example, I put so much pressure on myself to write my second play. A ridiculous amount of pressure. I'd spend days sat with my laptop being so angry with myself like "why can't you write? Why can't you do any-thing?". Whereas when I was messing about trying to come up with ideas, and just took the pressure off myself, suddenly I had the vision in my head of a stupid song, wrote that down. And the next thing you know, within two months, I'm about forty pages in and I'm gonna finish it! Compared to two years of trying to write something for glory with nothing to show. But now I've gone back to doing it because I enjoy it, for the love of it. I've stopped being a bellend! A watched pot never boils.

I feel like it's hard, because in this world we're taught that you have to succeed, you have to have money, you have to have a house. When you get to a certain age, it's gotta be like this. That really kills you. Especially acting-wise ... I'm 30 soon, and I think it kills me more because I'm still in the casting bracket for early twenties ... they won't let me act my age! I'm stuck with all the recent graduates who are hopeful with life – and I'm not! With all the pressure in society, I feel like I should be on TV by now, I should be achieving X, Y, Z by now. That version of me got nowhere. All I got was diagnoses. In my early twenties. I mean, much-needed diagnoses, hallelujah! But that's all I had to show for that pressure.

Whereas when I accepted it and just breathed and stopped putting so much pressure on myself, then I came out of that and started all my writing again. I started to do stand up. I then started to do some of my comedy characters. That's when my first play got written and I toured it. I'm so glad to be turning 30. My twenties were insecurities, being stuck in my conscious, figuring out my mental health, not accepting it. And I feel like in the end of my twenties I've accepted me. I'm quite happy to ask for space or turn down weekend plans because I would rather do nothing. I feel more grounded. So I'm very excited for the next part of my life, cause I feel like I lost the start of my twenties to mental health. I'm in a very different place now, it's like polar opposites – early twenties to end of twenties. Get to your end twenties, they're very fun!

### Impact of training in creative field

I wish I could lie and say I enjoyed going to university for acting. I learned things, sure. But uni wasn't a great place for me. I'd *just* turned 18, and I moved to the other side of the country from everyone. I needed to breathe. I was constantly told I wasn't going to cope there because of my anxiety. To be honest, fair dos. I thought I wouldn't either. I have issues with my eating that never got addressed when I was young, so I still really struggle with an undiagnosed eating disorder. When my anxiety is bad, that really grips me. So I had so much stuff going on.

I used to always get picked on at school, but I could laugh it off. Uni was the first time that I deliberately got set upon by a group of girls. That was horrendous. It was such a toxic environment where everyone thought they were the best thing there ever was, and they could speak to people a certain way. I only got bullied because I stuck up for someone. They didn't like that. I had three years of absolute hell.

I think training-wise, I met a few good people. I met a director that I absolutely adore. He does my plays with me. Do I think it was beneficial? No. Uni to me just reminds me of someone who was very ... unwell. It was a toxic environment to be in when I was so young. I was on beta blockers at one point ... it was not a highlight.

What I didn't realise until recently was how much I still clutch onto from uni. All the stuff that happened, stuff that now I need to unpick to be free from it. It was because they always used to hate the fact I can do serious acting, but I always used to get pushed to comedy more. I love comedy, and I love being daft. But when I used to get picked on and everything at uni, they used to say, "you're not a proper actor … you couldn't be a proper actor, you do stupid things". So I started to resent the thing that saved me my entire life, my humour.

I started to resent being the funny one. And I started to not want to be that any-more. I started to get angry with people when people would describe me – "ANON does comedy". No, I do other things. It was like my identity was gone. I didn't want to be the class clown, and I got really angry when I was doing it.

And it was only literally a few months ago when I met a casting director, and she said, "your CV is comedy, why is your showreel not showing your comedy characters?". I said "Well, I don't want people to think I'm taking the piss, wearing my wigs and doing my silly accents". She said "What … acting?". It was so stupid that her just saying that to me … "Ohhhh."

She said "You've been taught that doing your comedy is a lesser thing, and it's not. You hate yourself for doing the comedy, 'cause you even describe it as 'silly wigs' or 'doing something daft', whereas you've been on the front of Harrogate Comedy Festival with James Acaster. You've opened for the Frog and Bucket, you've won acting competitions doing comedy. You've got a really strong CV, but for some reason, you're embarrassed to be it". And that was only what … six months ago? Less than that. And then suddenly I just thought "my God, you're right … I hated that I was … I didn't want to be classed as comedy, whereas that's what saved me and that's what I am". And I shouldn't feel bad for it. So I feel like that was the last thing to unpick.

There's a lot of prejudice in acting. There's the Shakesperean actor, the working-class actor, the non-working-class actor. Everyone thinks they can do comedy and they can't. It's really hard. And if you can do comedy well, they just see you as just dicking about. But the worst thing is, because of my self-deprecating humour I'll be like "ha ha, yeah!". And … ahhh! I hate myself! Whereas now I'm starting to see, actually no. I am talented and skilled!

I shouldn't laugh! But no, I graduated when I was 20, it took my 9 years of achieving all this comedy stuff to just allow my showreel for casting directors to show me doing character comedy in my wigs. It's got me as an Essex psychic, and it's got me as an Yvette Fielding, and it's the first thing they'll see. Instead of being worried about whether I'll ever get cast in anything, I'm just like "this is what I do, if you enjoy it, there you go". I've stopped trying to over-psychoanalyse why I'm not getting brought in, am I being brought in, are you judging me for doing comedy, are you not?

Comedy saved me, and I feel like I was cruel to her. Because without realising the thing that was saving me and riding the success of it when it was successful, I was also embarrassed that people would just view me as the one who pisses about. Even though that's what saves me in life. I resented being seen as a joke. Which is a massive joke, really!

Cause I do clowning! You know when your life is a joke? This is it, this is like … what are you doing? I was embarrassed to be a clown, who specialises in clowning, who puts on clown shows, and then would be upset that people only saw me as a clown. Like … it makes no sense!

### Stigma

When we were writing a description of my play, I thought of The Muppets, hundred percent. It's one of the things that inspires me. I adore them. They're funny, funny guys. But did I write that to any of the theatres? … No. I looked at theatre companies that are nothing like what I do but they do some comedy sometimes, and put them down instead. I was still embarrassed for the humour I did, because the slapstick and the clowning comedy was still seen as below other comedy. Even though that's what I needed to breathe. So yeah. I would happily write for the Muppets.

I went to uni many moons ago now. There were a lot of horrible people in my year. When we were getting ready to leave uni (they don't do this anymore), the tutors got us all to line up, girls first, then the lads. Then they'd call out casting types that you would be. Like, "Who looks feeble? Who would look like 'the bitch'? Who would look like this? Who would look like that?" And then, one by one, the people would shout out a name of who would look like what. Then you'd be told "there you go, that is what your casting type is, cause that's how you look", and suddenly your identity changes. Some of the girls that were seen as being quite vulnerable were much happier than the girls that were classed as "the bitch". Whereas in reality, that is the wrong term, it's someone who looks like they've got a bit of fight in them, a bit gritty, probably lived a bit. But they were classed as that, and it was such a negative thing. Whereas the girls who were vulnerable thought they were like a Disney princess and happy in life.

What happened to me, in front of my entire year, was I always got picked to the top 3 in quite a lot of them, but then never got picked in the final bit. The person in charge then said, "you'll notice that ANON always gets to the final, but never wins". And people were like "oh yeah, yeah". And they then said that's because … well … "she's a bit of a schizo", are the words he used.

I've got an uncle who was schizophrenic, so I thought … "really?". But, he said "she's a bit of a schizo, cause she can play loads of different things, but isn't a main casting type. She doesn't have one". So I was the only person in my year to be told "you're a schizo and you don't have a casting type". That class ended, and I felt like a massive failure. What was going on? Body dysmorphia was coming in. "What's wrong with my face? Why don't I look right? Why can't I do this? Oh my god". Later I realised it meant I am a character actor, but that scene stuck in my mind. That I got called a schizo, who doesn't fit anything. I felt so lost. How do I enter a field where I don't belong? That was not a pleasant day.

### Everyday creativity

This is where my mind goes blank! Everyday creativity … obviously I do writing, but obviously that's a standard answer. Other creativity that I do … no, it's gonna sound stupid, is that stuff like playing with your hair or makeup, trying to make up new things. Or does that sound really daft?

Right, don't judge me. So I do stuff like that, I just play. I'll try things out. I would say another way I'm creative (that I'm hated for in my house) – I won't follow recipes, I wing it! I give it a little bit of this and a little bit of that, and I see what happens! Sometimes it works … majority times it doesn't. But I don't like being tied down to what I have to do. I like to be a bit spontaneous. And I definitely shouldn't, a lot of the time!

I feel like that's how I'm creative. I don't like being restricted; I test boundaries. Another thing that I think that I do … well it's more of a defensive thing … I speak in weird voices quite a lot. I do it at work as well. I think, whenever you meet me, I'm always the same as you know me. I don't have a filter. So I'll always do the strange voices, or if not I'll say things in German or Spanish. I suppose that's a little creative thing. My head's just like … quite content to always play and be doing daft voices, and I'll speak in different accents, and try and teach myself them. I entertain myself to get through the day. I think sometimes people where I work think that I'm really funny to be on shift with cause I'm entertaining them. In reality, I'm making myself laugh. To coast through that shift. It's just me making myself laugh for me!

| | |
|---|---|
| *Robert:* | ANON is not the first person to find connection between recovery and gelotology (the study of laughter). Increasingly, focus is being placed on understanding how laughter can benefit us mentally (Berger & Gonot-Schoupinsky, 2022). Similarly, the role of playfulness in wellbeing is being explored (Niklasson, 2022), which ANON seems to embody. Her creativity is rooted in a joyfulness, which shines through in how she speaks. When times are hard, this creativity is supressed, but when conscious of this, she can take the pressure off herself and find the joy again in time. I can still remember the excitable smile that crossed her face when she defined her creativity as play. By remaining in touch with the child within, she has been able to give voice and form to traumatic incidents from the past. To express them in ways that are joyful, and turn negative memories into positive experiences shared with and carried by the laughter of audiences and friends. |

### References

Berger, A. A., & Gonot-Schoupinsky, F. (2022). Humour and mental health: A case study of Arthur Asa Berger. *Mental Health and Social Inclusion*, *27*(*1*), 37–50. doi:10.1108/MHSI-08-2022-0051.

Niklasson, M. (2022). Mental health, art and creativity: Re-discover the child within. *Mental Health and Social Inclusion*, *26*(*3*), 292–298. doi:10.1108/MHSI-04-2022-0022.

# 10 StoryTeller – Anna Sexton

## Anna Sexton and Robert Hurst

> *Robert:* Jerome and Andrew had both previously come across Anna when she was working on her PhD project in information studies – she created a mental health recovery archive. Andrew was one of those interviewed for the project. We were keen to speak with somebody who had worked with recovery in an academic sense as well as having experienced mental health difficulties.
>
> I was very hopeful that our interview would be helpful to the research, but was blown away by Anna's story, and the ways that she was able to describe the interaction of her creativity and journey to me. For the final interview, this perfectly helped me to wrap up the ideas that had been developing.

**Anna's story**

I feel, in terms of my creativity, that it has helped, but also it's come back. For a while, I couldn't even be creative. I couldn't do anything. So that feels good, and I'm sure that's feeding back into things – being creative.

*Recovery*

This is a strange one for me, because having been involved with the term in an academic context during my PhD, I have an understanding of how it's been framed as "what a meaningful life means for you". Going back to feeling that your life is fulfilling. I've also, through all of that context, been aware of backlashes to the term recovery. How it's been co-opted by services. Aware of all the discussions and debates. But for me, personally, I don't think it's about recovering exactly who I was before I had psychosis. I don't think that is possible. It's a strange journey where I'm learning the ways in which it has impacted me and continues to impact me, and adjusting to that, to some extent. But I would go along with the idea that it's feeling that you are able to still … contribute. Feel relatively on top of things,

DOI: 10.4324/9781003319405-10

being normal. Able to function with family, with friends. With work. So yeah, I think it's being able to get to that place, I suppose.

Work has been the biggest challenge for me. Because I work as an academic, it's really demanding, and you are supposed to be brilliant. Mediocre isn't OK, you're supposed to be pumping out research articles and doing all of this stuff. Since I had psychosis, that simply hasn't been possible. I haven't had the mental faculties. I would describe what psychosis felt like to me as like a brain injury. Everything went. I couldn't concentrate, I couldn't focus properly afterwards. I think my brain was just trying to sort itself out again after this kind of explosion had happened, and so with work, sometimes I feel like I'm still just about clinging on. While I was trying to deal with the aftermath of psychosis and get back to normality.

With friends and family I feel my recovery has been really good, I feel that side of it has been great. But work is a lot more challenging, and I feel I'm a long way behind where work needs me to be. That's a source of constant anxiety, to be honest.

I suppose what I'm trying to say is that my recovery feels quite mixed. In one way, I do feel like my relationships with my family have healed, because obviously it has a big impact on everybody around you, and that has to be worked through. I feel like that's happened. But the work aspect feels really challenging.

I don't feel like I've recovered, and I have an anxiety that I just… won't be able to get back to where I need to be. I'm just about surviving! But that's all about the workplace, I would say. That's one of several different domains of recovery.

### Recovery with an extensive background knowledge

I haven't ever sat down and said to myself "OK, you're on a recovery journey, what does that mean for you?". I just haven't! It's just been about dealing with the aftermath of what I went through. Trying to work it all through. "Journey" makes it sound like it's a smooth, one-way process forward. It isn't. Things have come up at different points that I wasn't expecting.

Through my work with Dolly Sen, Andrew Voyce, Peter Bullimore, and Stuart Baker-Brown on the Recovery Archive project, I was obviously quite attuned to what a major mental health rupture is like for someone. I was very in touch with their stories. But it's a completely different thing to go through for yourself. There was a lot that I didn't know. I don't know how unique it is to me, but things like the physical symptoms that I had afterwards, I just wasn't expecting them. Like I have really bad tinnitus now. I'd never had that before.

So working through all of these different elements, some of them are psychical, some of them are trying to get your mental state back to where it needs to be, trying to deal with medication changes and that will set you back, or forward, and you never know whether you're on the right medication, or what impact that is having on you and whether it's a good thing or not. It hasn't been one-way traffic in terms of forward motion, at all.

Sometimes I would get ahead of myself, I would think I was well enough to do something, and then find that actually I wasn't quite ready for that. And that set me back. That's why I'm not sure I like the word journey. Because it becomes very one-way, and it's just not like that at all. It's unpredictable, I think, to a large degree.

I think because what I went through also coincided with the pandemic and lockdown, in a way that was helpful because I was able to make connections very slowly with people again. But then, there was a moment where I was suddenly meeting up with an old group of friends, who I hadn't seen for years. And rather than that being positive, for some reason it triggered things. Perhaps because memories were involved, it triggered something in me which was quite a big step back. I started to remember things that I had hallucinated in psychosis, that I'd buried. They came to the surface, and it was like I now have to deal with this, and that was… I wouldn't say it's a step back, but it was a new situation that I had to adjust to and work through, I would say.

Most of that recovery theory and knowledge went out of the window when it started to affect me. There were weird things that I remember from listening to Dolly and Stuart and Peter, which I could very much then resonate back to my experience of hallucinating. So there were points of connection between what they told me, and what they went through. But obviously it wasn't the same as their experience, it was different.

### CHIME

*Connectedness*

Well, I mean … that's been fundamental. I honestly believe that things would have been a lot worse had I not had the stability of the relationships that I have in my life. When I was very deep in psychosis, my partner made decisions for me which I know have really helped. He insisted that I wasn't taken anywhere, that I stayed at home, and that he would manage looking after me. I had to be with someone 24/7, it was that bad. But he made it very clear that I wasn't going anywhere. So initially, having that support around me was absolutely fundamental. Having that almost unconditional love to just go through what I needed to go through. Being surrounded by love, really. I am 100% that had I not had that, my recovery … I don't know where I'd be. Maybe still in psychosis, I don't know. I really feel for people that don't have that. There's lots of people that go through it without that around them. Knowing how horrendous it was, even *with* that, thinking about what it could be like without it is just … devastating.

*Hope*

I think it's very hard to be hopeful and optimistic after going through something like psychosis. And I still struggle with hope and optimism, because of the work anxiety. I always, in the back of my mind, think "what if I have to stop and give up work? What then?", and I can't then fully embrace this idea of hope or optimism, because of that anxiety. So I can see why the framework includes that. I think that's very difficult for people to be conditioned into thinking. "You need to be hopeful, you need to be optimistic".

Psychosis robbed me of so much. The way that it played out with the hallucinations, it took memories and entwined them with things that weren't real, and so you're left with an inner dialogue of "what's real, and where is the cut-off point?", having to reassess your own memories. When you're going through that process of trying to make sense of what has been traumatic and work it all out afterwards, it's very hard to sit there and feel particularly hopeful or optimistic.

At the moment I feel I'm very much between the past and the present, so looking ahead to the future seems very difficult.

*Identity*

I suppose what I would say is that I've got all of these complicated thoughts about work, but my family are the most important thing to me. So, healing with them has been fundamental. I would say my identity as someone who is married, and has children – that aspect of my identity I think has been extremely motivating and important. Because that has been the priority really. Making sure that I can function and give support to my children, and my partner. That I can be their mum, being there for them and supporting them has been really important. So that role has really pulled me forward in all this.

*Meaning*

This is where I would bring in some of the creative things that have been helpful. So, as I said, I couldn't really do anything creative for a long time. After I had psychosis, though I stopped hallucinating and I was back in reality, I was in very deep depression. Where I was just … I was sort of in reality, but I was not functioning or coping at all. I felt extremely numb from everything. Just couldn't feel anything, definitely felt completely hopeless. That lasted for quite a long time, that period of depression. And I would say that one of the things that has really helped with that has been when I began to be able to be creative again. So, although I was quite a prolific poet before psychosis, I actually haven't been able to go back to the poetry. I just still can't, I just … I just can't find the words at the moment.

But what I did do, which is through my mum, is I learned to sew. I'd never sewn anything before, except the odd crappy thing at school! What I do is nothing like my mum does, proper dressmaking. But I knew that I needed to be doing something that was creative but also that just occupied my mind. So, with sewing, I fell in love with the process of making. Sewing has so many different aspects to it. There's choosing the right fabric where you're thinking about the colours and how you're going to combine things. Then the pattern that you choose, and how you're gonna match that, or make alterations. And then there's the actual making process, which is obviously very tactile. You're using your hands, you're with materials, and you're also being highly productive. You've gotta concentrate and work out what's gonna go where, but at the end of it you've made something that you can wear! That's been, I think, really instrumental in me beginning to come out of the depression and beginning to feel better. And I think it is because it gave me a sense of … achievement?

While work doesn't feel great at the moment, yet here I am making something that I can wear or give to a friend. That has been really important. For a while, I just felt like my brain was never going to get back the ability to concentrate and function. So actually seeing that I could learn a new skill, that I could do it, using different parts of my brain, was a real confidence boost. That maybe my brain is going to be alright!

So I think it's a creative process, but it's also about the productiveness and the mindfulness element of it. If I'm working on that, it's enough of a challenge that my brain isn't going to go into an anxiety spiral, so it is keeping me on a material level of "I'm here, I'm sewing, my mind is occupied with things that feel positive".

So whereas poetry requires emotional creativity that I did not have, sewing is more of a tactile creativity.

*Empowerment*

I understand this as a feeling of agency. It has felt like a very wholesome thing. I'm not that big on social media really. But the sewing community is just all so positive, and people put up what they've made, and everybody is really lovely about it. It's probably one of the nicest online communities – there's no hate, it's all about what you have made, not what you look like. I would use the word "wholesome". It's given me access to expanding my social networks a little again. It feels very gentle and positive, I would say. So it's been good in terms of … I mean they're not friends or anything, but in terms of feeling that you are participating in a community, that's been positive.

I think I had this inbuilt feeling from the word go, just based on kind of the networks I built up during my PhD and listening to people who have gone through this sort of thing, that … just this phrase that Stuart would often say to me – "You need to be your own best doctor". You have to almost be in control of that. And I think, because of that, to some extent, I distanced myself from professional help. Although to be fair, not a lot was offered anyway!

But I haven't actively sought that, and it fell off very quickly anyway, really. To some extent I had this opinion that it was something that *I* needed to work through. And I suppose in a way that is a sort of feeling of empowerment. Although it doesn't necessarily always feel empowering, because you're struggling with so many things. But that sense of not relying on a professional to come and tell me how I should deal with it, necessarily.

I had kind of accepted subconsciously that it was something that I would have to work through and go through. But also, even in those initial conversations with professionals, I just felt that they would be no help whatsoever. The sorts of things that they were saying just wasn't worth at the time talking about it – about three people sat down with me with this model of resilience. The whole idea was "you have not been resilient", basically. "That is why you went through this, because a lot of people are really resilient – you're clearly not, and therefore you're here on this chart, and that's why you've gone through what you've gone through". Immediately I thought "that doesn't speak to me, I'm not interested in hearing that, that's just a load of nonsense as far as I'm concerned". You know, I don't lack resilience, I really don't. Anyone that has come out of psychosis in anything resembling human form has resilience.

It's things like that where I thought … you're not going to help me. I would describe to them, "I'm really struggling with concentration, and I'm really struggling with focus, and I feel like I've had a brain injury. My capacities are all over the place". And I was having physical symptoms, like I would sit in front of a screen and the words were spinning and I couldn't get my eyes to focus on the screen. And saying these things to them, it was like I was the first person who had experienced this. It was just so unhelpful.

Nobody was giving me anything helpful, so I just thought, "I'll just have to see if it gets better, and whether it improves". But your mind and body are connected, and I think if something has gone catastrophically wrong mentally, that then affects your sight and your ability to move in certain ways, or function. And so, looking back I'm like of course! I went through a majorly traumatic mental experience, and my whole body was in shock, you know? No wonder I had problems, like the tinnitus and the sight issues. Now, I can look back and I can understand it on my own terms.

I basically think my body went into complete shock, you know? Couldn't function. No professional said to me "at the moment everything is in shock, you need to give it a month ago and then see". Nobody said anything like that to me – I had to understand it for myself. It's disappointing for professionals to be taking something positive like resilience and looking at it in terms of deficit. As I said, anybody going through psychosis is resilient just by being, really.

### Creativity

Creativity can come in very many forms. I think it's that space to find ways to express yourself. It can be a tool for working through things, a tool for processing things. Interestingly, I haven't yet found that with poetry, but when the time's right, I feel like that will happen. It just isn't the right time for me right now. If I was gonna write poetry, because naturally you write from the self, it would involve thinking through what psychosis was and what it meant. And I just don't feel that I'm at a place where I want to dig into that, at this point. But at some point, I think that will happen, and that poetry will be a tool for working through another layer of it. I'm sure it will happen, but I'm just trusting my gut on things. I do think it will be a helpful tool when I am ready.

Whereas the sewing, it is tactile and mechanical, but it's not *just* that. It's also about self-expression. I think that's what creativity gives you. That ability to explore different sides of yourself that you want to work through in a safe way. And even things that seem quite mechanical aren't simply that. For a while all I could manage creatively after psychosis was painting-by-numbers. Somebody bought me a paint-by-numbers set, and I literally sat and would do that. Even that level of having your mind concentrating on something using colour, and then seeing a finished thing that is beautiful. Then, that mechanical creativity can be very beneficial. So I think there are different levels of creativity that different people can connect into, and each one has a potential benefit. And some of it is just ... because colour is beautiful. Colour helps the mind, it's therapeutic. Using colours in whatever way, even if it's just painting-by-numbers, is giving your mind something.

As well as the process, there is an aesthetic element to it. It's about connecting to that. In that when, I think that it can be a very deep tool for processing what you've been through. A way of helping you to make sense or put into place how you're going to interpret what you have experienced. Everybody will have a slightly different interpretation of what happened, like the reasons for it and why certain things occurred and what that then means for you going forward. And I think that sometimes engaging in a creative process around it can help you reach those conclusions.

It allows you to set out those experiences and look at them from a different angle. That is how creativity has played a role in my recovery. But what I would say is that I think it's important not to force it, either. So, for me, the poetry is not for now. I think it would be potentially dangerous to get somebody to do something they're just not in the right place for. That they're not ready for, that doesn't feel right to them.

It *has* to be that the person knows that this is something that they want to do, and that they wanna engage in. I guess the whole idea of creating models, I think it's great to have some kind of insight and some understanding into what will work for people, but as soon as it becomes a ... prescription, a general truth to must be followed, that can become destructive. The person has got to be ready for that. They've got to want to do it, or it's just not gonna work.

### Creativity as processing

Thinking about it, I did do some writing. As I said, I saw my friends, which brought back lots of memories and I ended up trying to work out then what was memory and what was psychotic hallucination. I went into a bit of a dip. And actually at that point, I wanted to help them to understand where I was at and what I was going through. So I did actually write to them. I did a few short pieces which were basically "this is what I've been through. This is what psychosis is like, and this is why I am where I am". So that's the only time that I've used writing as a form of processing for me, but also as a communication tool. To try and help them to understand where I was at. And I got to the end of doing that, and it was helpful, because it sorted through a few things for me. I was able to see where the memory stopped and where the psychosis kicked in. It was helpful even just to find the words to explain to someone who has got no concept of psychosis – "this is what it is like".

I used metaphor – if you imagine my brain as a filing cabinet, what psychosis has done is it has just ripped through all the files, pulled out all the papers and then jammed them back. My mind is trying to sort out where all of the papers actually go. It's trying to put everything back. And that's what it's done to my memories. And so, finding the words to explain this was important. I have done that, but then once I'd finished that, I knew I didn't want to do any more digging into what psychosis was like, or how I felt about it. That was enough. That's where I was at that point, so this is what I'm saying about listening to and trusting your gut about when to engage in something. Because I can see if I had kept digging, that might not have been helpful at that point. Self-awareness is needed.

To me the metaphor in itself was quite creative. It functioned as a kind of translation device, taking the experiences I had and putting them in a way that meant people who had no conceptualisation of what psychosis feels like could visualise it and put themselves in my shoes. It was writing about it in a creative way because I was trying to give them ways into the experience that would help them to connect to it or frame it.

It was cathartic. I was just … I do remember I was literally just … completely sobbing as I was writing it, because I think it was getting some things out that needed to come out at that particular time.

### Creative process

I don't have one! It's interesting because you have said "you're a highly creative person". I suppose I just don't really see myself in those terms at this point. So do I have a process? … No, I don't. I think I just trust that when I need to use a particular creative tool, I will use it.

Interestingly, the types of poems that I was writing before psychosis *were* about processing things that had happened in my life. So after my first son was born, I had quite bad post-natal depression. He's 16 now, and so when I was writing the poems it was many years after I had experienced that. But, I obviously needed to do something to try and make sense of what I had been through. That's what those poems were about, making sense of that rupture that we went through and what that meant … putting that in place and explaining it. So maybe in 10 years' time I will write some poems about psychosis! I think I'm quite slow at wanting to process these things.

I keep calling it a tool, creativity. But above all it feels to me like an instinct. I know within when I need to use it.

### Art versus creativity

I think there's a hesitation in saying "I'm a creative person". It's trying to distinguish between who you see as proper artists engaged in a process that will call themselves an "artist", and someone like me who … well, I do it for my own benefit internally. I don't call myself an "artist". I'm an amateur sewer and I'm an amateur poet. I suppose it is like that. But I *am* a creative person, in that colours are really important to me. The aesthetics of things are really important to me. So the way a room will make me feel because of the colours in it, or the way that things are arranged.

That's why I love fabric. Because of the colours and the patterns. That, to me, is a form of therapy. Looking through fabrics is therapeutic, because they're beautiful. And when you're engaging in anything that makes you feel that you're connecting to something that is beautiful, then that is quite therapeutic, I think. So, I am a creative person in that colour is important and self-expression is important. The dressmaking is about creating an aesthetic, so being creative in that way, I would say I *am* a creative person actually.

### Consuming creativity of others

This is a bit of a left-field example, but I mentioned being part of the sewing community online, and actually seeing what other people are producing and how they have creatively made something or hacked a pattern is amazing. I follow a lot of vintage sewers, so they're presenting in a 1940s style, with all of the gear, and it's all beautifully hand sewed. I find that really pleasurable, seeing what other people have made and what they've achieved! Engaging with it on an aesthetic level, and recreating it aesthetically.

It makes me feel happy, it makes me feel joyful. And again, the word I keep coming back to is wholesome – it's a really lovely thing!

Those groups are an oasis for me. I mean it's interesting, because art isn't always … beautiful. It can be very dark, and you can be expressing something very dark and horrible like psychosis. So … I can't think of any examples that I've seen like this, but I'm sure there are some very disturbing images, because I would describe psychosis as *literally* hell. I'm sure there are creative outputs that aren't aesthetically lovely, that explore very dark aspects of psychosis.

Maybe those are different kinds of creativity then. There's the wholesome kind which is aesthetically pleasing, then there's the dark and possibly more cathartic side of it.

### Originality

For me creativity definitely doesn't have to be original. The paint-by-numbers is literally paint-by-numbers. It's very restricted in terms of the input that you have to provide to make the output look a particular way. But with sewing, even if you're sewing a pattern, there's fabric choices to make, particular ways that you might adapt the pattern. So yes, you're taking something and you're using it as a guide, but to me the output is always *slightly* original, cause it's handmade. It's been created by someone who has made particular choices along the creative path.

I think what I'm saying is that even something that is completely "unoriginal", like if you and I paint the same paint-by-numbers they're going to look pretty much identical … That's still a creative act, to me. Because, yes, you're being completely directed, but to me creativity is about engaging with the with the act of making a thing. The process.

### Creativity within a discipline

In my particular field, I feel that there's scope for my students to be exploring more creatively than we allow them to. I have actually been thinking about this quite a lot, because going back to my poetry, I lecture in archives and records management. I do have a set of poems that are exploring aspects of what records mean to people and why they're important, and how that connects to identity and memory. And I feel like my students could equally be engaging with the concept quite creatively, and thinking about it quite creatively, but the course is not designed to enable them to express their theoretical thoughts or their distinctions between different parts of the discourse in a creative way. I think that's a shame. I'm sure not all students would want to do it that way, but some of them I think do. So I think creativity is … to some extent shut out in my particular area of work.

### Impact of stifled creativity

For me, my creativity not being accessible to me was one indicator that what I'd gone through was very severe. The fact that my body and mind had shut down that ability, alongside a number of others, to me it just shows the level of shock that I was experiencing having gone through that.

I *tried* lots of different things. After the paint-by-numbers, I knew that creativity was important, and I needed to reconnect. I was trying different things. So I sat down and tried to write some poetry. No words came. I just couldn't connect into that. So then I tried just painting with watercolours. And interestingly, I just picked a thing off the internet, and again I wasn't doing an original painting, I was just copying something.

I was in a very deep depression at that point, and it was the effort of getting the paints down, choosing something to paint. I can remember it all just feeling completely overwhelming. I remember saying to myself "just try and get to the end of the painting".

I got to the end of that painting, and I felt completely numb. I just … closed down the picture, put the book away. I found the painting just after Christmas. I looked at it and I thought… "That's actually quite a good painting that I did!". I felt no connection whatsoever to it at the time that I made it. But I've actually framed it, and it's in our living room! I put it up on the wall, because to me it symbolised how even when I was totally numb, and wasn't even really connecting to this painting, I still made something beautiful.

### Meanings of creativity changing through time

Do you see what I mean? To me, even when you are absolutely on your knees and you feel dreadful, there is still potential in that. I think that's what this painting symbolises to me. That's why it went on the wall, because if I go through any more dark places (let's hope I don't), I have all these reminders around me now that even when you're absolutely at your worst, there is still a spark in there. You've just got to find it again.

There are things in there that *will* come out again.

The painting itself, it doesn't really matter whether it's brilliant or not, it's what it now means to me that is so important.

### Understanding the creative instinct

It's hard to say how I *knew* that I needed to be creative … how *did* I know? I suppose it's just knowing that it's a part of you that you know is important, both in terms of marking where you are, but also as a tool for getting you somewhere. I guess it's all the times where I've been creative in the past, and reaped the psychological benefit of that. So I knew that it could be a path to something, I suppose, from previous experience.

### Creativity as museum metaphor

Sense-making is very important, isn't it? We all want those ways to curate ourselves. Being creative is one of the ways of doing that. Well, it's probably the only way, because I can't think of how you would create your life story without it having an element of creativity in it somewhere. That ability to curate your story in the way that you want to curate it, having those markers of what that means. Like that picture, it marks something for me, something important. That's why it went on the wall. Having that ability to curate your story is huge.

And interestingly, another thing I haven't mentioned … I also felt it was really important to get a tattoo to mark what I'd been through in psychosis. I've got one on my leg, and that was a creative process, even though somebody else produced the artwork. Because I had a very clear vision, an idea of exactly how this tattoo had to look. And each of the elements of it symbolise something for me. So there's a lighthouse, there's … this is gonna sound crazy! The lighthouse is my partner, basically. That symbolises my partner, and the sun behind the lighthouse is my eldest son. And then there's rocks, and there's a … a blue-tongued skink. My son has a blue-tongued skink called Dustin. So that represents my youngest son.

Each of the images represents what pulled me through psychosis, which is essentially my family. I felt it was very important to have this actually *on* my body. Because if I ever go back into psychosis again, I want something on my body which will help me to remember the things that will pull me out again. So yes it's somebody else's artwork, but it was a creative act on my part. Choosing symbols for yourself of things that are really deeply meaningful also feels like an act of protection. This might sound crazy, but that's how I see it. It's protecting me for the future as well.

This is basically what I teach in my job. History in an official sense is a curated story, usually through the eyes of the victor. The person who controls the archive controls the story. So having the ability to control what you might call your own creative collection or archive, is a way of putting yourself in order again. After something like psychosis that is really important, I think.

*Everyday creativity*

I would say that almost every choice you make has a creative element. So for example, I dress according to my mood. I'm very much affected by mood when I'm sort of choosing what I want to wear. Even those aesthetic choices in how you're gonna dress or how you're gonna present are creative acts.

I hate cooking, though! I don't get any creative feelings from cooking at all, I literally follow the recipe and get something on the table that people can eat! So that's not particularly creative for me. But for other people I could totally see how it could be creative.

Then I suppose there are intentionally creative things, where you know that you are doing something for a creative purpose. So at the moment the overwhelming one for me is sewing, but I paint, poetry has been big at particular points. Writing is creative … So even in my job, when you're writing something which is weaving together perspectives, that is creative. So I work with lots of small moments of creativity. Where you're pulling together ideas, you're presenting them, whether that's in a lecture or in an article you're trying to write or whatever it is. There are certainly creative aspects to that. And then there's being intentionally creative, where you're sitting down to be creative, because you want to be.

I think anything that involves imagination and sense-making, even subconsciously, is creative. It's like a kind of background creativity, which compliments the more intentional creativity.

| | |
|---|---|
| *Robert:* | This conversation with Anna felt like a perfect way to round off the interviews. Anna spoke clearly and eloquently about her experiences, and pulled together a lot of the ideas that had been coming up for me during this stage of the research. Her feelings about the importance of colour and beauty in particular struck a chord with me – it summed up how intangible our emotions and feelings can be at times. When we have a bad day, being around something bright or something that gives us a sense of wonder can turn the day around. This is something that I do not believe can be truly measured with instruments and questionnaires. Hence the need to understand stories in the detail we have in these StoryTeller chapters. |

# 11   Andrew's story

*Andrew Voyce*

I will discuss in this chapter how creative activities have helped me on my recovery journey. How they have helped me to find a place in the world.

I have to say that I would have liked to have produced art and other material that would have been valued for its stand-alone merit. Instead, my creative output has served the purpose of telling an untold story, which has enabled me to move on from difficult episodes. My creative output includes cartoons, music, and written texts.

There is a practical application for creativity in sharing narratives with others, and enabling others to create their narratives. Being able to create stories for others has allowed me to embark on a parallel journey through technology, which I have endeavoured to keep simple, accessible and affordable. A personally meaningful reference that the alienation of the schizophrenic involves submission to delusions (Rhodes, 2000) restates the power of living with false beliefs, and I have somehow escaped that, to record in retrospect the detail of psychosis. This I have done through creation and with catharsis.

## Paranoid schizophrenia and me

Before reading any further, the reader may wish to know that I have paranoid schizophrenia. Though, despite my surname, I do not hear voices. I have had my days, when psychotic, which have been occupied by false beliefs. I was asked by a psychiatrist once if I heard voices, and my reply was that I heard my parents and grandparents who are Voyces, was that what the gentleman meant? That is after all my name. So no, I do not hear voices. Rather, I have strange beliefs when psychotic. But yes, I do respond to medication (Steingard, 2014).

My current prescription of atypical antipsychotic tablets dates back 20 years, and prior to that I took daily medication of typical tablets for 10 years. I am not amongst the number whose symptoms remain unaffected by medication. I have always responded to antipsychotic medication, the big difference being that I have not had unacceptable side effects from my current prescription of tablets. Unacceptable side effects led to me escaping supervision to avoid that medication by injection, the driver for 20 years as a revolving door patient with multiple admissions. I am therefore compliant because the therapeutic effect of tablets is

DOI: 10.4324/9781003319405-11

different from the therapeutic effect of injections. Those 30 years of therapeutic support from medication with acceptable side effects have coincided with years without inpatient episodes, without arrest, without homelessness, and during that time I have not felt paranoid or suffered from delusions, although I usually lack insight into my symptoms. It may even be possible to say that by me taking medication, I have ceased to trouble the criminal justice system.

I need also to mention that during those 30 years since my last hospitalisation and the advent of community care, I have had weekly counselling which has complemented effective medication. I am not among the number of schizophrenics, who may or may not hear voices, who are given over to futile and failed treatment. I am happy with a life on medication. Because there are people with psychosis who do not respond to medication, this can inform a body of opinion against all medication, backed up by respected academics and speakers, who even deny that there is such a thing as schizophrenia. The following chapter is of me leading a journey of recovery from a devastating period of psychosis.

I object to being taken as a deluded fool by those who deny the existence of psychotic illness, or who deny that medication can only be an untoward tool. I also give respect to those who hear voices and who find ways of coping with voices without medication and who do not accept that voice hearing should be diagnosed as schizophrenia.

## Diagnosis

I have a diagnosis of paranoid schizophrenia, and as this allows the description of false beliefs, non-consensual views of reality and delusions, I can accept that I am included among the population of people with schizophrenia in the UK. To be described as a paranoid schizophrenic can actually be helpful (Steingard, 2014). Sometimes I joke that if the men in white coats come looking for me, I will be looking for the fire escape, and furthermore I refuse to go back to basket weaving in occupational therapy.

I have come a long way from those dark places, and demonstrate that I am in fact capable of much more than weaving baskets, sewing soft toys, and doing menial tasks in industrial therapy units. I have emerged from those days (which totalled twenty years), and highlight the futility of that time; since then I have obtained a bachelor's degree with honours, a master's degree in social policy, successfully run a social enterprise for three years, written articles for academic journals, delivered lectures to university students, and commissioned a website with my creative efforts detailing a historic record of my journey. It's a pity that some of this could not have been organised when I was in my twenties rather than my seventies.

## Mental health recovery

There are some theoretical propositions on recovery that I have come across or that I have created myself which are intuitive to me. The concepts of alienation, Keynesian economics, and social inclusion are among those talking points which

I pick up quite easily. I have self-discovered the value of personal narrative and before I identified it as autoethnography, I had reached my own definition for such methodology (Voyce, 2019). These are the ideas which I am familiar with.

I did not discover recovery in mental health by myself, I was introduced to it during the first years of the twenty-first century. Publications such as *Mental Health Recovery Heroes Past and Present* (Davies et al., 2011) and *Psychosis: Stories of Recovery and Hope* (Cordle et al., 2011) were very influential for me. I took on the notion that recovery in mental health is not necessarily about getting better, or getting back to a place where you were before, and neither is it the same as the 12-step programme for recovery from substance abuse. Recovery in mental health involves hope and perhaps also a degree of heroism.

The definition of recovery highlighting hope is person-centred, it is about the service user and clearly puts the recovery model at odds with the medical model. To focus on the individual's strengths and resilience is fundamentally not to say that a simple prescription of antipsychotic medication is all that's needed for a person with schizophrenia. The medical model treats mental illness as such, and I have lost many years while psychiatric authorities have attempted to fix me as if I had a broken arm or pneumonia with medical interventions.

The search continues for a link between brain activity, the effect of medication, and genetic links to the development of schizophrenia. Clearly this spells out a divide between those who prescribe medication as the only necessity (and who are perplexed when it does not work) and those who seek to find the unique individual within. My struggle with the psychiatric system was around medication, and the unwillingness for responsible clinicians to remove me from drugs that caused side effects that were so severe that a life on the streets as a vagrant was preferable to compliance.

When I was last discharged from a mental hospital at the age of 40, I emerged into the world of community care. Crucially, I had negotiated to have medication by tablet which caused acceptable side effects (Voyce, 2018b). This happy coincidence of no more asylum bed waiting for me, medication with which I complied, and resources in the community, coincided with the advent of my recovery. Mental health care was reaching new ground. This was indeed a guiding vision, and I was to find out what this vision meant. What it looked like in practice.

**Recovery and the medical model**

As remarked elsewhere in this book, there is no overarching definition of recovery in mental health. There are common themes however which can inform mental health service delivery. Shepherd et al. (2008) identified their principles of recovery as moving away from looking at symptoms, deficits and pathology, and towards a search for meaning and strengths. I find it no problem to identify with this paradigm. For me, hope in the sense of having agency and a degree of control and choice are essential for successful community living. At the advent of community care, such aspects of recovery were essential for people leaving institutions after many years, such as myself. We had to re-learn skills to cope with life as newly empowered, and discharged from the "cradle-to-grave" mental hospitals.

As well as this meaning and engagement with life, I have a comfortable identity after moving on from being a chronic mental patient. Sometimes just saying that amazes me and puts my journey into a perspective. It does not seem possible that a life which included living rough in cars and bus shelters and incurring criminality has turned around, and that I am now secure in the belief that the revolving door will no longer be part of my life. And yet, those years have given way to a life which indeed includes hope, a satisfactory identity, meaning in my life where I can be considered as a responsible adult with ability to influence or change.

Drennan and Alred (2012) seek to distance hope from pathology in their support for recovery-focussed service delivery. The authors show a support for anti-psychiatry and identify recovery as a political model. Clearly this carries on the polemic with the medical model, although Secure Recovery (Drennan & Alred, 2012) includes clinical recovery along with functional, social and personal recovery in their model. For these authors, it is necessary to be able to complete living tasks, to have social connections and for recovery to have a personal meaning. It is necessary to have hope for these outcomes.

## CHIME and hope

Let me reflect on two further descriptions of recovery. Hope, identity, and personal responsibility are key for Watson and Meddings (2019). Hope is the common factor for many descriptions of recovery. Indeed, Watson and Meddings maintain that medical treatment in mental health can be as damaging as symptoms themselves. They cite the top-down critical movement of the anti-psychiatrists, and the bottom-up direction of the service user movement, which have brought about change and a recovery focus in mental health care. My caution (Voyce, 2020) and that of Shepherd et al. (2008), and Drennan and Alred (2012) is that therapeutic recovery needs to be in place.

The gift of hope, and an identity beyond that of "mental illness", is essential to recognise. Because we recognise the limits of the medical model does not mean that it is appropriate to discard the place for effective interventions of medication and talking therapies. That may deprive some of a recovery journey. In this context, talking therapies can be taken to include the coping mechanisms of the Hearing Voices Network and the National Paranoia Network. Of course to be able to assume personal responsibility can lead to social integration, and goes alongside a happy identity that is not that of dependant psychiatric patient. I have to say my doubts are when symptoms or disclosure lead to lack of respect and failure to be included as a socially responsible person. Rightly or wrongly, this is the case, and Allport's (1954) ladder of discrimination may unfortunately become a factor in how people with mental health challenges are viewed and stigmatised.

CHIME is more than a literature review. Along with elements of recovery that others include (hope, a satisfactory identity and a meaningful life), CHIME includes connectedness and empowerment. I have found that helpful relationships with family (which have been restored), work, and other people have become protective factors. Hope goes along with empowerment to enable an identity that I and others who know me can share. So, along with these descriptors of models of recovery which are more than the medical model, goes a dialogue around the ownership of recovery.

There is no literature to rival personal narratives of recovery. For me personally, the collateral damage of pre-recovery-era psychosis has included the loss of my house. I believe that today's person-centred and recovery-oriented services may have meant that I would have remained a property owner had they been in place when I was last psychotic. Certainly I have spent the last 30 years in the community, mostly in my own rented home albeit rented.

### Creativity for me

What then of creativity in my recovery journey? Creativity sustained me in several ways during 25 years as a dependent community care patient, until I reached retirement age and perversely became independent through part-time work and the receipt of my state pension. Many sources give four outcomes for those with schizophrenia:

- premature death, often by suicide (I had three clear suicide attempts during my prodromal and institutionalised years);
- needing or being required to accept constant support (I spent time in mental wards, and council, church and therapeutic hostels);
- to be "somewhere in-between"; and
- to be recovered.

Well, I can say that I have paid all my bills for six years without recourse to means-tested benefits (Living with Schizophrenia, n.d.; National Institute for Health and Care Excellence, n.d.). This "in-between time" occupied those years from 1991 to 2016 when I was a dependent community care recipient, and it was good that resources were in place for me. Creativity played a huge part in my use of statutory services.

I count as my creativity: art, writing, making music, growing flowers, creating a business entity, and indeed going on a recovery journey. That 25-year period in-between psychosis and chronic association with the asylum system was a remarkable journey. I took encouragement in being involved in the service user movement. I was empowered to write my story. I took it upon myself to take the initiative in growing a garden at the day centre. I was on a recovery journey from dependence and institutionalisation to freedom and choice, meaningful engagement with society as other people live it. This was a journey to a place where those above would count me as recovered. I travelled on a recovery journey from being looked after to independence.

When I wrote down my story, I felt like I was beginning to get my life back. It was indeed helpful that my caregivers at the day centre read and appreciated my writing. It was also helpful that staff members invested time to type up my handwritten notes. On taking these notes which were on floppy discs (remember them?) to the local business centre for them to prepare paper booklets, which I paid for, I owned my narrative in more ways than one. I keenly listened to people who were able to help me to make full screen colour images of my narrative. As well as making images in the programme Paint, I picked up how to use PowerPoint and lo and behold I had semi-animation. It became apparent that caregivers of all occupations (including artists) were supportive of what I was doing. These relationships sustained and empowered me. I knew telling my story in words and pictures was doing me good. I felt I was breaking ground, and I was convinced that I was creating innovation and uniqueness in the digital age.

## Creativity and recovery

Creativity means I can share my journey with others of a like mind, for example by illustrating my story with a talk and presentation. This I find to be immensely creative, and it has sustained me for the years since I was last in psychiatric care. If my narrative is not about recovery and C-CHIME, what is it about? I am convinced that Repper and Perkins (2003) have the journey understood correctly - that stability through interventions can be built on to produce a rounded person. In some little way I have road-tested that notion, and have been empowered by creativity.

There is a notion that madness and genius are linked – that there is a fine line between the two. There is an implication that such as Nobel Prize mathematician John Nash's schizophrenia was linked to his genius at problem-solving. Perhaps he would not have had amazing qualities in maths had he not also been a sufferer of psychotic symptoms. His brilliant mind naturally tipped from genius to mad person. As for art, a famous example is Vincent van Gogh. His genius with colour and the paint brush existed alongside an unstable mind, leading to spells in asylums and personal self-harm. The two were co-existent.

To be sure, I am not comparing my creative outlet to that of Nash's academia, or van Gogh's artwork. I have some prowess at both academic and artistic endeavour, and both involve a creative element. No matter what subject one studies at higher level, including advanced mathematics, one cannot just be marked as 10 out of 10. Higher academia requires the mark of the individual, one cannot obtain an award for being "correct" – one has to be creative and individual.

What I wish to say on creativity and my output is that I acknowledge that my creations are far from perfect. I have not produced "top quality" material; it has never been spoken of as such. I would have loved for my artwork to be greeted as unique and worthy of comparison with van Gogh. It clearly is not so. I would have loved for my digital book of personal narrative to have gone viral. It has remained in a quiet corner of the internet. So, no, my work has not met with acclaim and clamour. That outcome, I have long realised, will not come about. But what I have succeeded in doing is to tell a story in many ways: looking at various aspects of personal narrative, reworking, reauthoring, and using a variety of platforms. This, to me, is where I am at. This is the basis of the mechanics of my creativity.

I once saw a Tweet (now deleted) that summed this up for me. It read along the lines of "The greatest aspect of recovery is insight". It doesn't cure or solve the condition, but it does a damn good job of making the navigation of life easier. It allows you to educate people on your condition and advocate for yourself. Managing decisive moments. In the same way that McManus and Carson (2012), Repper and Perkins (2003), and others explain, once the symptoms of psychosis are under control, insight can follow and this can result in self-expression to enable catharsis, a creative process.

**Reworking and co-production**

Sharing and collaboration are features of modern creativity. Sampling and remixing in music demonstrate creative re-working well. Elements can be taken from one source and modified into something vastly changed. For example, Puff Daddy's "I'll Be Missing You" (which I like) samples the riff from the Police's "Every Breath You Take" (which I do not like).

I have always found it good to collaborate when producing a creative effort. In the summer of 2022, I produced a zine with Recovery Partners of Sussex and their mentors – Ant, Jo and Lucy. *Alienation Handbook* was an empowering project and allowed me expression. There is a paper version, as well as an electronic version.

Possibly for me, my most significant collaboration has been *Side Effects* (Voyce et al., 2012) – a graphic book about my life journey. This samples my digital cartoons which were made into a storyline by Hannah Cordle and the artwork was reworked by Oivind Hovland. A re-working and a co-production. These are major features of my creative environment, and my work with Professor Carson also falls into that category, with several collaborative autoethnographies to our names (Hopkinson et al., 2021; Voyce & Carson, 2020).

**Community care**

The Hearing Voices Network (2012) asked the question "whose recovery is it anyway?" Is this for the benefit of the service users or the staff? Are service users being led into a false sense of security where recovery is the disguise for service reduction? Certainly in the latter part of that 25-year period where I received community care, my much-needed day care support where I had practised art, learned how to make computer art, ran a user-led computer art group, and had worked in the lovely garden, changed radically. The garden is now locked up, vandalised and abandoned. As I understand it there are very few and restricted therapeutic or creative groups that take place there. The 24/7, 365 days-a-year service, where people could count on support at those dreadful lonely times including Christmas, has been reduced to a few hours during weekdays only. The guise is "signposting". This process cannot be ignored, it needs to be acknowledged and has been accelerated and exacerbated by the mantra of austerity. There is something indeed to the critical point of view of "whose recovery is it anyway?".

Perhaps Judi Chamberlin (2012) had a point when she wrote that separative services where non-patients and professionals are excluded are the only valid configurations for the true service user movement. Equality with non-patients and professionals is not good enough, and neither is partnership in name only, for Judi. This is a creative and political point to reach. And yet my personal recovery has proceeded in this environment that could be portrayed as compromised by some.

When I began to write down my story, the manager of the day centre said to me, "you could not have done this a few years ago". She was right. As I became secure that psychosis would not return and that I would not again end up in an institution, I also was able to look back on my last five years of schizophrenic homelessness and to recognise my thoughts for what they were: false beliefs, delusions, and a non-consensual view of reality. I realised that I did indeed believe that people from Newcastle were doing untoward things in southern universities and police stations. Another psychotic belief which had bugged me for many years was that I had a transmitter in my artificial leg that told the traffic where I was, and that the traffic was following me around. I believed that the Russians were about to arrive. I believed that Morse code signalling was going on wherever I went, it was everywhere. I was convinced that my identity had been stolen.

In writing my story, I was at last able to say: "I recognise that my thoughts were overcome by false beliefs during my last period of psychosis, and I now recognise this as a period of delusionary beliefs, and I have written them down to share with others". The benefit of this creativity was fourfold. In writing the false beliefs that I had, there were moments that can only be described as therapeutic, as is found by many creative people. Along with that, the recognition that these beliefs I had were non-consensual with other people's perceptions resulted in a cathartic experience - a cleansing. As well as this moving on, there was also a tangible object, a book, which I could share with other people such as family, friends and caregivers. And most importantly of all, I was telling my story from my point of view with my words and pictures, it was not someone else's version of who I am. I am not "narratively entrapped" (Grant & Zeeman, 2012); I am narratively free. It has given me a sense of identity beyond that of a psychotic person or a psychiatric patient. There is power in re-authoring a personal narrative. McIlveen (2008) writes of the transformative effect of autoethnographic creation, and my cartoons and other output have helped me to leave behind a life and identity as a revolving door psychiatric patient.

My personal narrative was typed up by a member of staff at the day centre, and I was able to have books made at the local business centre with this digital format. I have reworked this to create *The Durham Light and Other Stories* (Voyce, 2018a). Back in the 1990s, I began to make digital images with the help of staff at the day centre. I graduated to make full colour slides of episodes in the old asylum system, and to draw pictures illustrating my times of psychosis and what went through my head. I combined these Paint images into PowerPoint format, and they became sequential art which can be found online (Voyce, n.d.). I selected titles such as "The Good Old Days" and "Get Well Soon" to express the irony of my 20 lost years as a revolving door patient.

Digital technology  As well as personally experiencing the fourfold effect of therapy (catharsis, recognition, having a tangible object, and ownership of my story), I was able to encourage others to tell their story. In keeping with the Internet principles of accessibility, democracy and empowerment, I used quality and affordable methods to produce paper books of personal narrative for others in both graphic and text form. As Bill Gates is said to have put it: "The Internet is becoming the town square for the global village of tomorrow". I am proud to have produced personal narratives for a number of people, and quite often this process has accompanied the journey of mental health service users from inpatient care to step down into the community.

As well as finding my voice through creativity it is helpful to update, and make relevant, the media I choose. The cartoons I have created on my asylum experiences are surely more accessible because of their format. The story can be understood in digital pictures without necessarily needing to read the speech bubbles. In fact, the cartoons can be scrolled through as a piece of sequential art (a means of graphic storytelling), and a famous example is that of the Bayeux Tapestry. My sequential offerings have been reworked into forms such as my graphic novel, *Side Effects*. I am inspired by cartoon forms such as Manga, and can see the relevance of graphic storytelling in gaming. I am very taken by the graphics of comics, government leaflets, and the reworking possible through digital programmes. There is a link between style, media, and storytelling which is of a younger generation, and which is accessible.

## Conclusion

My recovery journey has been facilitated by access to creativity over 25 years from the psychiatric ward to independent living. Yes, creativity has allowed me to express myself and I would not have wished for anything else on that journey. I have lived through an era which epitomised the advent of the recovery model and the nadir of the medical model. I have had epiphany moments, perhaps the most important of which was the writing of my personal narrative. This process is what has been valuable to me, rather than having created a celebrated work of art. I have, like Gordon McManus, "written myself better" (McManus & Carson, 2012).

## References

Allport, G. (1954). *The nature of prejudice*. Addison Wesley.
Chamberlin, J. (2012). *On our own*. National Empowerment Center.
Cordle, H., Fradgley, J., Carson, J., Holloway, F., & Richards, P. (Eds.) (2011). *Psychosis: Stories of recovery and hope*. Quay Books.
Davies, S., Wakely, E., Morgan, S., & Carson, J. (Eds.) (2011). *Mental health recovery heroes past and present*. Pavilion Publishing.
Drennan, G., & Alred, D. (Eds.). (2012). *Secure recovery*. Routledge.
Grant, A. J., & Zeeman, L. (2012). Whose story is it? An autoethnography concerning narrative identity. *Qualitative Report, 17*(*36*), 1–12. https://eric.ed.gov/?id=EJ989819.

Hearing Voices Network. (2012). Whose recovery is it anyway?. www.hearing-voices.org/events/whose-recovery-is-it-anyway/.

Hopkinson P., Voyce A., & Carson, J. (2021). Syd Barrett took a left turn and never came back, Andrew Voyce did. Why? *Mental Health and Social Inclusion, 25*(*4*), 385–395. doi:10.1108/MHSI-06-2021-0031.

Living with Schizophrenia. (n.d.) Can you recover from schizophrenia? https://livingwith schizophreniauk.org/information-sheets/can-you-recover-from-schizophrenia/.

McIlveen, P. (2008). Autoethnography as a method for reflexive research and practice in vocational psychology. *Australian Journal of Career Development, 17*(*2*), 13–20. doi:10.1177/103841620801700204.

McManus, G., & Carson, J. (2012). *From communism to schizophrenia and beyond: One man's long march to recovery*. Whiting and Birch.

National Institute for Health and Care Excellence. (n.d.). What is the course and prognosis of psychosis? https://cks.nice.org.uk/topics/psychosis-schizophrenia/background-info rmation/course-prognosis/.

Repper, J., & Perkins, R. (2003). *Social inclusion and recovery*. Bailliere Tindall.

Rhodes, C. (2000). *Outsider art*. Thames and Hudson.

Shepherd, G., Boardman, J. & Slade, M. (2008). Making recovery a reality [policy paper]. https://mentalhealthrecoverystories.hscni.net/wp-content/uploads/2014/01/Making-recovery-a-reality-policy.pdf.

Steingard, S. (2014). The problems of non-consensual reality. www.madinamerica.com/2014/09/problems-non-consensual-reality.

Voyce, A. (2018a). *The Durham Light and other stories*. Chipmunkapublishing.

Voyce, A. (2018b). The established state and patient X's rebellion. *Mental Health and Social Inclusion, 22*(*3*), 128–133. doi:10.1108/MHSI-02-2018-0003.

Voyce, A. (2019). Unintentional participant observation: A research method to inform peer support in mental health?. *Mental Health and Social Inclusion, 23*(*2*), 81–85. doi:10.1108/MHSI-01-2019-0001.

Voyce, A. (2020). Two narratives: Recovery journeys in mental health. *Mental Health and Social Inclusion, 24*(*2*), 105–110. doi:10.1108/MHSI-03-2020-0011.

Voyce, A. (n.d.). Andrew Voyce. www.slideshare.net/AndrewsAsylumLife.

Voyce, A., & Carson, J. (2020). Our lives in three parts: An autoethnographic account of two undergraduates and their respective psychiatric careers. *Mental Health and Social Inclusion, 24*(*4*), 197–205. doi:10.1108/MHSI-07-2020-0045.

Voyce, A., Cordle, H., & Hovland, I. (2012). *Side effects*. South London and Maudsley NHS Foundation Trust.

Watson, E., & Meddings, S. (2019). *Peer support in mental health*. Red Globe Press.

# 12 A new model of creativity in recovery and C-CHIME

*Robert Hurst*

One of the first things to say is that, based on what the StoryTellers have told us, perhaps creativity isn't strictly related only to recovery. Rather, it seems that creativity is an urge, a desire, that pulls you through dark days. It is fuelled by darkness and light, and through play an individual can use the catharsis of creativity as a kind of stabiliser. A way to safely explore, and make something bright.

There is more nuance to this than "creativity can help people along in recovery". I think that, through the process of conducting this research, I have felt that *everybody* uses creativity in some way to heal. For those we describe as "in recovery", this of course becomes more pertinent.

This chapter will outline the results of the qualitative analysis performed on the transcripts of my interviews with Jo, Michelle, Peter, ANON and Anna. This includes three themes (each with sub-themes), a model of creativity in recovery, and a conceptualisation of how creativity would work as a sixth dimension to the CHIME framework. These will be illustrated using quotes from the original interview transcripts.

As established in the introduction, both recovery and creativity are terms without definitive definitions. As such, it is important to begin by attempting to define both in regard to the five StoryTellers' experiences.

## Recovery

A key aspect of recovery for the StoryTellers is that it is different for everybody.

> Everyone's got their own unique journey along the way.
>
> (Michelle)

As well as being "unique", recovery is very much personal, "individual" (Jo). It is something that can only be done by the person in recovery.

> You just need to figure out your own path with it.
>
> (ANON)

DOI: 10.4324/9781003319405-12

I … accepted subconsciously that it was something that *I* would have to work through.

(Anna)

Here, emphasis was on "I", highlighting a sense that professional help was not always useful in recovery.

Not a lot [of professional help] was offered anyway.

(Anna)

Another issue was that the StoryTellers felt that in many ways recovery was exclusively owned by mental health professionals, and that they perhaps did not have a say in their own recovery.

[recovery has] been … colonised, in some ways.

(Peter)

The word recovery itself was held in question, with each StoryTeller having words that they preferred to use, such as "navigate" (ANON) and "discovery" (Peter). For Jo, no word was needed at all.

To recover from something, it suggests that you've completely got over it. … I've always felt it's the wrong term to use. … You don't even have to call it anything.

(Jo)

This sense that there are expectations around "recovery" was felt throughout the interviews, and personal barometers for recovery were discussed.

Recovery for me is having a quality of life that is acceptable to me.

(Peter)

Everyone talked about a need to be heard, for people to listen to their recovery experiences.

I dunno if [psychiatrists] listen as much as they should.

(Michelle)

Being listened to was important, as recovery "can't be defined by measured outcomes" (Peter), and "is a journey not a destination" (Michelle). Although Anna did not agree with this terminology.

I'm not sure I like the word journey. Because it becomes very one-way and, it's just not like that at all. … it's unpredictable.

(Anna)

This unpredictability means that, more than following a model, adapting to what is in front of you is something many of the StoryTellers preferred to see as a way of continuing in recovery.

> Recovery to me means learning to navigate your normality.
>
> (ANON)

> it was a new situation that I had to adjust and work through.
>
> (Anna)

This is important to note, as while time played some role in recovery ("there's … stages", Michelle), it was seen as something that required effort, with words like "work" (Peter, ANON, Anna) being used to describe recovery.

> people need to be proactive.
>
> (Michelle)

To summarise, for our StoryTellers recovery has been a very personal journey that requires a great deal of effort. While there is no ultimate destination, it is a mindset of adapting to each new scenario as it arises and finding an acceptable quality of life. The language and approach of professionals could be unhelpful, leaving StoryTellers feeling unheard.

## Creativity

The most striking thing to emerge from the interviews was the existential way that creativity was described. Particularly from Jo, who described it as an "essence", and "*the* all-encompassing force of the universe". Others also spoke in almost spiritual terms about creativity.

> music is … like my soul.
>
> (Michelle)

This tied in with the way in which creativity seemed to almost be an unconscious instinct.

> all I can do is create from the urges I get.
>
> (Jo)

"Urge" seems an appropriate word, as creativity would appear very quickly, and be experienced as an in-the-moment phenomenon.

I've got to get [an idea written down] there and then.

(Peter)

Of course, not all creativity is like this, sometimes it is necessary to create something, perhaps for work.

I put so much pressure on myself to write my second play.

(ANON)

This is experienced differently for ANON from in-the-moment creativity.

I'd spend days ... being so angry with myself ... whereas when I was messing about trying to come up with ideas, and just took the pressure off myself, ... suddenly I had the vision in my head of a stupid song.

(ANON)

"Suddenly" is a key word here, emphasising the instantaneousness of creativity versus the "days" of trying to make something. These are seemingly distinct experiences, well distinguished as "creating" in the moment, "producing" by need. This fits the suggestion of Anna that "there are different levels of creativity that different people can connect into". Not all creativity is the same and can operate in different ways depending on context.

However, a more universal feature of creativity identified in the analysis is that everything created is unique. Because "every moment is completely new" (Jo), each thing made is therefore different from anything that has come before.

even if you're sewing a pattern, ... it's the fabric choices that you've made, it's the ways that you might adapt that pattern. So ..., yes you're taking something and you're using it, but to me, the output is always slightly original.

(Anna)

So even when using pre-existing elements, the resulting combination is new.

I often take components from different places, and use them, maybe with a sprinkle of something else usually from up there [gesturing to the heavens], to present something in a different way.

(Jo)

Unlike some definitions of creativity explored in Chapter 4, with the StoryTellers it did not feel as though something had to be brand-new to have been creative.

if you and I paint the same paint-by-numbers they're going to look pretty much identical ... That's still a creative act.

(Anna)

As such, creativity "can come in very many forms" (Anna).

> anything that comes out of me, has been created.
>
> (Jo)

All of the StoryTellers were able to identify their own Little-C everyday creativity. This ranged from packing a shopping bag efficiently (Peter) to making colleagues laugh (ANON) to choosing an outfit for the day (Anna) and yoga (Michelle). Anna identified that we can be creative throughout our normal day without knowing it, but also "intentionally creative" (Anna) when "you sit down to be creative because you want to be" (Anna). This normality enforces the idea that creativity should not be restricted to the arts:

> I think we can *all* be creative. I think we can all be artistic, there's probably different levels of how the art will look.
>
> (Peter)

This highlights that art is dependent upon value judgements of the quality. However, creativity itself is not subject to this, it is for *"all"* of us, as Peter emphasised. This is important, as it seems that this confusion of art and creativity leads to a disenfranchisement from being creative.

*Robert:*   We specifically asked you to interview today because Andrew has identified you as a really creative person ...

*Anna:*   [laughing] Has he? That's very sweet of him! [laughing]

The way that Anna instinctively laughed, showing disbelief at the idea of being a creative person, was striking. As the interview went on, however, she was able to disentangle her creativity from the value judgement of "art".

> there's sort of hesitation in saying... "I'm a creative person" ... trying to distinguish between who you see as "proper artists" engaged in a process ..., and someone like me ... I'm an amateur sewer and I'm an amateur poet. I suppose it is like that. But I am a creative person.
>
> (Anna)

While assigning value judgements of "amateur" to her creative output, she was still able to identify as creative. Seeing oneself as creative can be difficult, as creativity and the self are often intertwined.

> I would say [creativity] is me ... there's no separation between me and an artifact that has come from me.
>
> (Jo)

As such, it is unsurprising that creativity *did* play a role in the recovery journeys of The StoryTellers.

*Table 12.1* Themes of group experiences of creativity in mental health recovery.

| Superordinate themes | Psychological process | Sense-making | Social |
|---|---|---|---|
| Subordinate themes | Instinctive<br>Engaging<br>Cathartic | Ordering chaos<br>Imbuing meaning<br>Finding meaning | Pressures<br>Conditions<br>Escape |

## Creativity *in* recovery

Three themes were identified around how the five StoryTellers experienced creativity in recovery – as a psychological process, as sense-making and socially. Each of these had three sub-themes (see Table 12.1).

## Theme 1: psychological process

I think it helped me get through so much, developing creativity.

(ANON)

This theme encompasses the ways in which StoryTellers experienced creativity psychologically as a process, and how that impacted them in their recovery journey. This is divided into three sub-themes – instinctive, engaging, cathartic. The creative process could be all three of these things. Supporting quotes for each of the subthemes are presented in Table 12.2.

### Sub-theme 1.1: instinctive

How creativity came to be used in recovery seemed to be instinctive to StoryTellers. A "need" (Anna) or compulsion to be creative was described. When pushed on how she knew that creativity was important, Anna was unsure, highlighting the instinctive nature of this drive. It is not necessarily a conscious decision to be creative to feel better, but an impulse.

This creative process is felt as being forward-moving. It acknowledges the past for inspiration, "marks" the present, and pushes you forward as a "tool for getting you somewhere" (Anna). Even at low points, being creative is indicative that recovery is possible – creativity symbolises "potential", giving hope. That this seems to come instinctively is a sign of the importance of the role of creativity in recovery.

Peter demonstrated this instinctiveness in an interesting way – as a voice hearer, he has noticed that one of his voices embodies his creativity, is his "creative side" (Peter). ANON described a similar embodiment of creativity, as a side of their that was a natural reaction against feeling unwell. The forward-momentum nature of creativity means once it is used successfully, it becomes a vital part of moving along in recovery. In terms of moving forwards in a recovery journey, when you

*Table 12.2* Quotes for psychological process sub-themes.

| Psychological process sub-themes | Supporting quotes |
| --- | --- |
| Instinctive | "I … knew that I needed to be doing something that was creative" (Anna)<br>"I *had* to be creative" (Michelle)<br>"So mental health tries to restrict my head, …, but then the creative side of me wants to play (ANON)<br>"[my creativity had] been locked away by all those negative feelings." (Peter) |
| Engaging | "It's enough of a challenge that my brain isn't going to go into an anxiety spiral, so it is … keeping me on a material level of "I'm here, I'm sewing, I'm… my mind is occupied with things that feel positive" (Anna)<br>"I think the creativity allowed me to… on my recovery I wasn't wallowing as much when I *could* breathe" (ANON)<br>"Seeing that I could learn a new skill, and that I could do it … was a real confidence boost" (Anna) |
| Cathartic | "I do remember I was literally just… completely sobbing as I was writing it, cause I think it was like getting some things out that needed to come out at that particular time. So yeah, it was cathartic." (Anna)<br>"I got that little poison out again." (ANON)<br>"sharing it that way, it gets it out of you as well, … the guilt and things like that." (Peter) |

"can't stop" (ANON), creativity is a vehicle for momentum, for "carrying on" (ANON).

This is also reflected in experiences of creativity feeling stifled. Being unable to allow this creative impulse was "devastating" (Peter) and felt like "drowning" (Michelle). It had a huge psychological impact which was felt in almost a spiritual way, in the "soul" (Michelle). So, while creativity can act to improve recovery, if you are feeling unwell, the creative instinct can be dulled.

Negative psychological experiences were described as overwhelming the instinctive creativity, "locking" it away (Peter). This indicates that a certain level of recovery is required before the instinct begins, and that the creative instinct does not automatically start upon feeling unwell. Rather, it takes time for the mind to unconsciously lead you to creativity in order to move forward. For Anna, she was still struggling to find the words to write poetry despite having done so prolifically before experiencing psychosis.

Trying to force this creativity can have a negative effect. In trying to do so, you can bring on negative thoughts and impact your recovery negatively. Therefore, it is important to "trust" (Anna) the instinctive nature of recovery. The felt sense from the interviews was that following these instincts on when to be intentionally creative leads to the best outcomes.

### Sub-theme 1.2: Engaging

Anna in particular identified that when being creative, you are "engaging with the … act of making" (Anna). This side of creativity involved engaging the mind in things outside of any mental difficulties, and finding a sense of purpose in producing something. Anna also identified a "mindfulness" element to this process, that by using materials in a tactile way, it kept her on "a material level" in the present moment.

This indicates that when involved in a creative process, one can escape difficulties or anxieties. This was also seen in Michelle's account of editing a film, where she "used to sit there for 12 hours a day editing" (Michelle), lost in the process for large amount of time because it gave her "a focus" (Michelle). Peter reported a similar phenomenon when being creative in the kitchen. When focussed in this way, it is harder to be engulfed by negative thoughts, to "wallow" (ANON), allowing chance to "breathe".

For some on a recovery journey, being engaged in something positive can seem impossible. Achieving this through creativity can boost self-belief and confidence. Another benefit is the innate value of surrounding yourself with beauty.

"Engaging in anything that makes you feel that you're connecting to something that is beautiful, then that is… quite therapeutic" (Anna)

### Sub-theme 1.3: cathartic

One of the outcomes of engaging in a creative process was a sense of catharsis, having released bad feelings from within. The StoryTellers indicated that being creative is a means to letting out negative feelings such as "guilt" (Peter), which felt like "poison" (ANON), and that this leads to releasing emotions. From here, positive emotions can come into the process too, with StoryTellers using words like "joy" and "pleasure" to describe their experiences of being creative.

A sense of control can also be gained from creativity. Peter described how he thinks creatively about how to best wash the floors in his apartment, as this gives him a feeling of personal control, which is important in recovery. Having made something can be a way of finding control, and gives a sense of "achievement" (Anna) which can be "instrumental" in recovery. ANON said something similar, that if they had not been able to get catharsis from expressing their life experiences in a creative way, "I don't think my recovery would be what it is" (ANON).

Having experienced this sense of catharsis throughout life is important, as it seemed to train the creative instinct for Anna, meaning that when she found herself in recovery, she could turn to creativity knowing that it would be a "tool for processing" (Anna) what had happened.

However, catharsis was not always found from creativity. Michelle described it as a "double-edged sword".

> I've worked so so hard and got so mentally ill over my film, I have to be careful about creativity.
>
> (Michelle)

This shows that if one tries to put too much into creativity, tries to force it, one risks setting oneself back in recovery. This again emphasises the importance of trusting instincts around creativity, and that "you've got to know your limitations" (Michelle) when it comes to being intentionally creative within recovery.

## Theme 2: sense-making

> For me, meaning is … living, I think.
>
> (Michelle)

This quote emphasises the importance of making sense of your experiences. This theme includes how creativity was used by StoryTellers to find meaning in their experiences, how meaning was imbued into their creations, and how finding meaning in creations played a role in recovery. Supporting quotes for each of the subthemes are presented in Table 12.3.

### Sub-theme 2.1: ordering chaos

The creative process involves turning a variety of emotions, experiences and inspirations into something tangible. As Jo put it, creativity is an "essence", and "you can manifest the form that you wish from that essence" (Jo). In terms of recovery, that can mean understanding what you have been through. These experiences are not straightforward; indeed they are often "chaotic" (Michelle).

In the context of recovery, creativity is making sense out of "chaotic" experiences, making them into something "meaningful" (Michelle) and "interpreting why you have experienced them" (Anna). Creativity was seen as a "safe way" to explore the past, and to reframe yourself in a more positive light.

This ability to control the narrative was explained well in a metaphor by Jo. In the metaphor, creations are "artifacts", which you can then collect and look back on in your own "museum" which marks "evolutionary process" (Jo). It is important to acknowledge that the narrative created and ordered through these narratives belongs to the individual. It gives ownership to the person in recovery.

Having a narrative is seen as allowing one to have an overview of where they have come from, where they are now and where they would like to go. This narrative does not have to be factual. Anna was helpful to speak to about this metaphor, as a lecturer in archivism – "the person who controls the archive controls the story" (Anna).

*Table 12.3* Quotes for Sense-making sub-themes.

| Sense-making sub-themes | Supporting quotes |
| --- | --- |
| Ordering chaos | "[Creativity has] allowed me, when I was ready, to … not view myself as being broken" (ANON)<br>"you'll never understand a person's experience without a comprehensive narrative" (Peter)<br>"Having a … means of putting yourself in order again, after something like psychosis is really really important, I think." (Anna)<br>"I need to get rid of them. It's my past, it's gone. And er… some memories, I don't want to be reminded of." (Peter) |
| Imbuing meaning | "I've used it actually, over the years, my creativity in visual form and in written form to express myself" (Jo)<br>"But by drawing it, then [art therapist] could say to me 'is this what you're telling me?'. And then I could say 'yes'. So that for me was really important." (Peter)<br>"Everyone else will laugh at it, and I'll be laughing, but I know the undercurrent of it is my childhood trauma. [I'm saying] 'this is how I cope'" (ANON)<br>"I can get unwell if I … look too much into myself, about my mental illness, I'm not good" (Michelle) |
| Finding meaning | "If … it was 'the only interpretation', then we'd never put it in the gallery, show it off or anything" (Jo)<br>"I've always liked the work of Van Gogh. Cause I knew he was a voice hearer, and I know there was a story behind all the pictures." (Peter)<br>"If I ever go back into psychosis again, I want something on my body which will help me to kind of remember the things that will pull me out again" (Anna) |

Therefore, the person in recovery is able to curate their artifacts and create a narrative that means something to them. After "chaotic" experiences, this longitudinal ordering is a way to frame what has happened.

Anna stressed the importance of this in recovery, that through creating order from chaos, you can have a clearer sense of identity. "Curation" is also a key word in this metaphor, as one has the ability to keep only what is meaningful, to choose what stays in the story.

For example, Peter kept only a select few paintings that he created early in his recovery. Here, Peter demonstrates how he actively curated his own "museum" of artifacts – some paintings symbolised a low point in recovery, which Peter was "disappointed" with. As this was not a part of the narrative which Peter was curating, he threw those paintings away.

History in an official sense is a curated story, usually through the eyes of the victor.

(Anna)

The "victor" controls the story. By actively curating a narrative through creative artifacts, one puts oneself in the position of victor within one's own recovery journey.

### Sub-theme 2.2: imbuing meaning

Creativity can be a method of expressing meaningful things to others. In the context of art therapy, this can be helpful in processing trauma from childhood. It is a way of expressing difficult things through symbols rather than words, as Peter described.

Being heard was identified as an important part of recovery, and sometimes creativity is the language through which those in recovery communicate. Having those experiences understood is important, and is something that Michelle "wanted".

This desire for people to understand can only be done through creativity – finding the right words to describe these experiences to people itself requires creativity (Peter, Anna). This sharing is not necessarily overt. For ANON, a comedic actor and writer, this meant sharing experiences in a humorous way. Their father passed away during their childhood, and they find that they always put a joke in their writing about death. This is a way of making meaning from the traumatic experience and turning the negative into something positive.

This imbuing of meaning is important to ANON, it is a "coping" strategy, and also becomes a force for good, allowing people to "laugh". This process may happen unconsciously at times too – Peter described noticing themes relevant to his recovery in his book only after it had been published. He was "expressing things" about himself that he was not aware of at the time of writing. Expression and meaning imbuing were still taking place, but at the time Peter did not understand the relevance.

Once a work is shared, how others understand meaning in the artifact, whether intentional or unconscious meanings, is up to them. As Jo said, it is "not her business" how others interpret her work. Sharing lived experience requires creativity from both the sharer and from the listener.

Trying to look too far inwards in order to imbue meaning into creations is not always a good idea, however. Michelle described feeling "unwell" if she looked too deeply within. This demonstrates that digging too deep could hinder recovery. Rather, it is best as suggested earlier to trust instincts on how far to look.

ANON described not "touching on" everything in their mind when creating, and "joking about it" to avoid considering the true sadness of it. Again, this shows the instinctive nature of creativity, and that the personal narrative crafted must be appropriate for oneself.

### Sub-theme 2.3: finding meaning

Often we find meaning in others' creations. Humans ascribe meaning to everything, and these will not always be the intended meaning which the creator imbued their work with. However, this ability to find your own meanings in a work is what makes them special. As such, to share a creation requires "vulnerability" (Jo). While this can be "scary" (Michelle), sharing experiences is important within recovery, as discussed. Finding meanings within the creations of others can also be beneficial.

Michelle compared music to "eating and drinking", showing the vital nature of it for her. For ANON, the worlds created by Jim Henson were "1000%" a fundamental element of their recovery journey due to the escapism provided. However, meaning can be found in shared experience expressed through creativity.

Peter found meaning in the narratives behind the pictures painted by Van Gogh, as they bear some similarity to his own. Interestingly, some StoryTellers found new meanings while looking back on their own "artifacts". These meaningful interpretations were possible even if they were not intentionally imbued during the making process. Peter painted his own version of Van Gogh's sunflowers in art therapy, and this hangs on his wall at home because it "shows me how far I've come", and acts as "a driving force" in his continuing recovery journey.

Anna had a similar story – she got a tattoo which included elements that symbolised important people in their life. Having these images psychically on her body "feels like an act of protection". More than simply understanding experiences, this demonstrates how a sense of meaning can be "protective", a lifeline that will hopefully pull forwards in recovery.

## Theme 3: social

A flower can't help growing. It doesn't limit itself. They don't put any conditions on it. They grow because it's natural, they don't question it. They don't question things like we do. We're more, I think, used (or conditioned) to limiting ourselves.

(Jo)

While natural creativity may instinctively rise "like a flower", social elements will have an impact on this. This theme examines how social pressures and conditions impacted recovery and creativity, and how creativity provided a form of escape from these. Supporting quotes for each of the subthemes are presented in Table 12.4.

### Sub-theme 3.1: pressures

When sharing creations, the work is viewed and appraised critically by others, through the lens of societal expectations. Anticipating this judgement can limit creativity, which in turn can impact recovery.

Jo stated that her life would have been "very different" had her creativity not been "suppressed". She felt that once this negative critique is passed on "artifacts", one is "turned off" (Jo) from one's creative instinct, and this "just takes the life out of you" (Jo). The language here is strong, indicating that for Jo it is a matter of importance that creativity be allowed to be "free" (Jo).

*Table 12.4* Quotes for social sub-themes.

| Social sub-themes | Supporting quotes |
| --- | --- |
| Pressures | "If my natural creativity hadn't been suppressed from an early age, … my life journey would have been very different" (Jo)<br>"[As an actor] you're always persecuted for how you might sound, how you might look, and everything" (ANON)<br>"If I'm creative …, sometimes it makes me anxious" (Michelle)<br>"There was so much pressure to do it, my creativity stopped" (ANON).<br>"I find that really pleasurable, seeing what other people have made and what they've… achieved" (Anna) |
| Conditions | "It's being in the environment, I suppose isn't it? A creative environment, you know. The office job ain't gonna do it" (Michelle)<br>"I can't be creative… if my mental health is really bad… [shakes head]" (ANON)<br>"Cause for a while, I couldn't even be creative. … that feels good, and … that's feeding back into things – being creative." (Anna) |
| Escape | "I used to do a lot of gymnastics, and I felt that gave me a sense of freedom. I didn't feel trapped in this body. You know, I felt that I was free like the wind, and I think that, that's creativity" (Michelle)<br>"And it was my little thing, it was my thing that no one could…My private thing, you can't tell me what to do. I'm empowered to do it myself." (Michelle)<br>"I had to escape the world I was in, and I went to Jim Henson, and I went to Muppet Treasure Island" (ANON) |

One domain where creativity is suppressed is through professions – Michelle and ANON both worked within creative industries as a filmmaker and actor respectively. Rather than being able to be *more* creative through their profession, they felt that boundaries and expectations within those industries created pressure. This can lead to negative psychological impacts, which set recovery back.

Michelle felt excluded from the filmmaking community, due to being "too old". This resulted in her creativity "making me feel even worse", due to the pressure that she put herself under to achieve in the field. For Michelle, this need to "fit in" means that at times feeling creative makes her "anxious".

Here, the natural creative instinct is inhibited by social expectations. When the "artifact" created is not up to these social and internalised standards, it can lead to "frustration" (Michelle), can make creativity "punishing … torturous" (Michelle). This can lead to "jealousy" (ANON), which turns the creativity competitive.

This constant creative comparison can create a sense of self-"hatred" (ANON), and not one of catharsis as can arise from more instinctive creativity.

The pressures leave a person disempowered from their own creative passions. ANON described how the social pressures in acting made them embarrassed about the creativity they produce, even though that creativity is what had helped them through recovery.

This is not to say creativity need be *completely* free from social boxes. Creating requires "some structure, obviously" (Michelle) – a movie requires a camera, music requires an instrument, etc. By its nature, creativity requires a "form" (Jo), and these forms act as a common language, through which we can communicate. However, high expectations and negative critique can impact recovery and then creativity itself.

However, this pressure does not always lead to a negative outcome. A change of mindset can ease the inhibition of creativity.

But the thing with success is how you view it.

(ANON)

If you lower your internal expectations, decide to be less swayed by what is expected of you externally, creativity can become motivated.

I always want to make people feel happy.

(ANON)

As ANON says here, their intention is to achieve some social good through their creativity. In this way, the social pressure can become a drive, a motivation.

Additionally, some social spaces are supportive and seeing others creating and being praised for their creativity serves to motivate internal creativity. Anna found this on a "wholesome" online sewing group. This implies that safe environments do exist where creativity can be shared without harsh critique, and where seeing others achieve drives you to create in order to also "achieve".

### Sub-theme 3.2: conditions

As well as social expectations, social conditions can limit how creative a person can be. ANON spoke of their university degree as a "toxic environment" (ANON), which stifled their creativity.

Michelle echoed the word "environment", showing that this is a key element of creativity – being in the wrong environment "ain't gonna do it". In her office job, Michelle reported feeling that her "soul was … drowning" (Michelle) due to not being able to express creativity, and this led to "suddenly" feeling "mentally ill" (Michelle). This echoes the phenomenon noted in the "pressures" subtheme, where not all jobs inspire creativity ("it's *very* competitive", ANON). However, it is not as simple as then leaving this "toxic" environment.

Socio-economic factors impact the ability to sit down and be intentionally creative. Primarily, Michelle needed money in order to survive. Her psychological needs, her "soul", had to be put on hold by necessity. Longer creative projects especially require time and energy – resources.

Peter took "15 years to write" his book. Lockdown provided an opportunity and need to "be doing something". This demonstrates that when resources *are* available, creativity can flow much more easily. This is an important consideration with recovery. One of the conditions that needs to be right for creativity to be beneficial is to be at an appropriate point in recovery.

ANON indicated that when mental health is "bad", creativity is stifled. This becomes a "vicious cycle" (ANON), where frustration at the unproductivity feeds into making the mental health worse. When creativity *can* flow, StoryTellers reported feeling better, and vice versa.

This virtuous cycle, where feeling more well leads to more creativity leads to feeling better still is important to note. Is it possible to achieve this intentionally? Actively creating some conditions for yourself can give some structure, without too much pressure, which helps motivate creativity.

> And sometimes it is good to sit down and say ... I've got from five till seven [to] do it.
>
> (Michelle)

Here, Michelle demonstrates how setting time-based conditions helped to push her instinctive creativity – she spoke about needing to plan a film shoot, but then creating the "best shot of the film" spontaneously on set. This shows that by making yourself comfortable (in this case by being well-prepared), there is room for creativity to be more instinctive, more free.

This is relevant to recovery, because by learning where the boundaries lie, and how far you can push yourself, it could be possible to create a condition for yourself to express creativity and aid recovery. When inhibitions are lowered, StoryTellers reported creativity flowing better – whether that be through drinking alcohol (Michelle), being off heavy medication (Peter) or blocking out the world with music in headphones (ANON). Knowing the personal limits of this is important, however.

Anna explained how she felt writing poetry would happen "when the time is right". The conditions need to be "right", otherwise she knows that she may do more harm than good in terms of recovery.

### Sub-theme 3.3: escape

One way that creativity impacted the social dimensions of StoryTellers' lives was the opportunity to briefly escape from it. This is in line with Jo's description of creativity as being inherently "free" (Jo). Michelle described being driven to creativity as it offered "comfort" (Michelle). This idea of creativity as being "free", releasing one from the constraints of the world is beneficial to recovery.

Michelle described the "private" nature of her creativity as "empowering", it allowed the creativity to be instinctive and provide a "comfort", away from the issues in her life.

Similarly, for ANON, the created worlds of The Muppets provided a way to "escape the world" and find "enjoyment" (ANON). Having experienced this escape, ANON then went on to use their own creativity to try to provide escape for others. They try "to make you forget about everything that has happened." (ANON).

ANON reaped the benefits of this escapism recovery-wise, and decided to pay it forward in the hopes of providing a similar escape to others. Getting this sense of meaning from their creativity has aided their recovery.

## Model of creativity in recovery

Below are two models of creativity in recovery, as interpreted from the data. Figure 12.1 shows a straightforward linear model of creativity (see Figure 12.1)

Here, chaotic, existential experiences are filtered through creativity, after which they become ordered, meaningful and tangible artifacts. This process, as discussed, is beneficial to the recovery journey. It is an engaged state, where one is engaging with one's inner self. However, this is an idealised model, and creativity cannot always be experienced in this linear way. Figure 12.2 incorporates a social dimension.

Here, social factors such as pressures and conditions interrupt the flow of experience to artifact. They cause frustration, and creativity can become stuck in a frustrated loop, taking longer to (or never) become an artifact. This frustration can come in at any stage of the creative process between the instinct and the finished artifact. These frustrations feed back into the creativity, and either inhibit or frustrate it. The ways in which this can happen, and the resulting impact, have been outlined in the "social" theme.

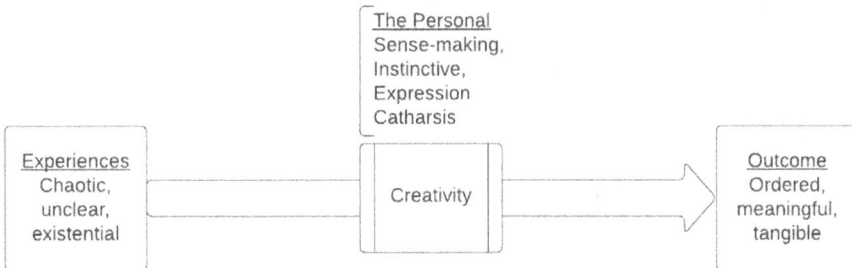

*Figure 12.1* Model of creativity in recovery.

Created by author.

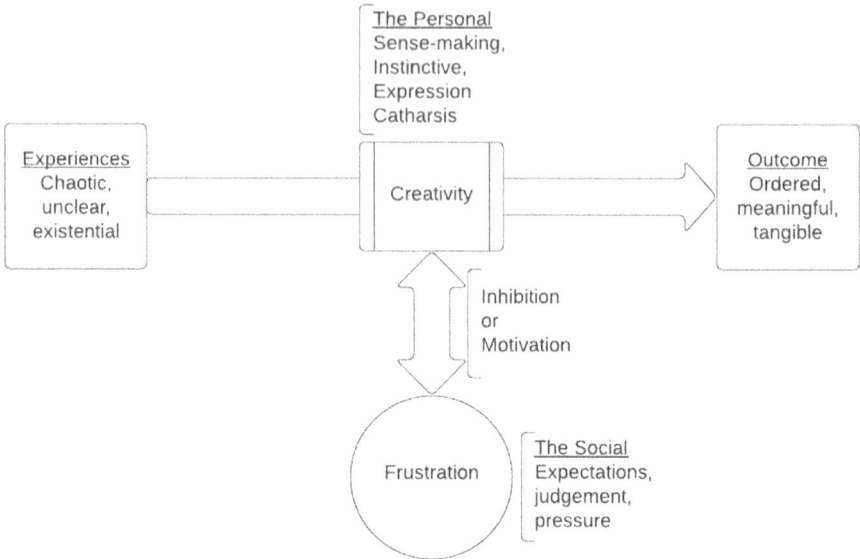

*Figure 12.2* Model of creativity in recovery, including social factors.

Created by author.


## C-CHIME

While it was one of the aims of the study to explore the suggestion that creativity should be added to the CHIME framework, this could not be done within the inter-pretative phenomenological analysis (IPA). As CHIME already exists as a construct, using that framework as the basis for analysis would not have been allowing for natural interpretations of the StoryTellers' experiences. However, through the analysis process, a way of understanding these experiences of creativity in relation to the other CHIME dimensions temporally became apparent. A table representing how creativity interacted with the five CHIME dimensions in the past, present and future within the dataset is presented in Table 12.5.

From our StoryTellers we begin to see that creativity is an intrinsic force. It interacts with the outside world for good (catharsis, expression) and bad (pressure, rejection). It is, however, something within all people. Expression of this being allowed, whether by the self or by others, is seen as something that moves a person closer to wellbeing. As per Rogers, an individual's uniqueness being allowed to be expressed brings a person closer to their authentic self (identity). It can create connections with others through sharing (connectedness). Creative artifacts can create a feeling that the self has moved from a bad place to a better one (empower-ment), that this is likely to happen again (hope). Having a passion expressed through creativity, whether the ultimate intent with that is merely for fun in the process or fame from the product, gives a sense of purpose (meaning).

*Table 12.5* StoryTellers' experiences of creativity in recovery, in relation to the five dimensions of CHIME across the past, present and future.

|  | Past | Present | Future |
|---|---|---|---|
| Connectedness | Creativity helped maintain connections when times were difficult. | Communication tool to help others understand your current experience. | Plans to share work with others, potentially making new connections or enriching current ones. |
| Hope | Being able to look back on creations from when most unwell, providing hope that things will not get that bad again. | Creating and experiencing a hopeful affect. | Creating in the hope of one day sharing it with others. |
| Identity | Able to look back and chart evolution of self through artifacts. | Able to express internal self, create expressed identity. | Being able to share experiences, breaking down stigma over time. |
| Meaning | Finding new meanings in artifacts. Making sense of experiences earlier in recovery. | Making sense of experiences in the here-and-now. Creating snapshots of current self, imbuing with meaning, future artifact. | Having an ongoing project provides a sense of purpose. Meanings will change over time. |
| Empowerment | Empowering to see the progress made when looking back at artifacts. | To be in creative state is to be present, in-the-moment. Mindful. Sense of control. | Sense that through creativity, can maintain wellness and continue in recovery. |

With this in mind, we suggest the addition of creativity to the existing CHIME framework to create C-CHIME. Our belief is that creativity can be just as important in the recovery journey as the other CHIME dimensions. While further work would be needed to cement this in evidence, we feel that a C-CHIME framework can be a useful supplement to CHIME for the time being – something for mental health recovery researchers to consider.

## Conclusions

Something that was felt throughout the process was the absolute vitality of creativity for recovery. So much so that the absence of creative energy can serve as a warning sign.

[creativity going away] was one other indicator that … what I'd gone through was very severe.

(Anna)

It is hard to sum up in short quotes something that was much more overarching across all five, full interviews as well as the myriad conversations I have had with people in my years researching this topic. However, the below encapsulate this fundamentality for creativity in recovery.

Comedy saved me.

(ANON)

You've got to be creative to survive. … Without creativity, I'd find it hard to be here today.

(Peter)

The language here implies life or death. This is why it is important to understand the role of creativity in recovery. Because it "saves".

# 13  Conclusions

*Robert Hurst, Andrew Voyce, and Jerome Carson*

This final chapter will summarise the discussions raised so far throughout this book. Findings from the work will be recapped, with implications and suggestions for future research made. Finally, each of the three co-authors will present their takeaways from the book.

## Findings

This project has aimed to evaluate the current state of play in psychological literature about the role of creativity in mental health recovery, and challenge this through interviews with people that have lived experience. Their stories have been analysed by Robert to suggest a new model of creativity in recovery.

In Chapter 1, we outlined some historic precedents for creativity as a means to wellbeing even in dire circumstances, before explaining the key terms and premise for the book. Jerome gave readers a sense of how the concept of mental health recovery has developed through the years in Chapter 2, before Robert focussed on the CHIME (connectedness, hope, identity, meaning, empowerment; Leamy et al., 2011) framework in particular in Chapter 3. Robert then evaluated the concept of creativity within psychology in Chapter 4, arguing that there is a confusion between scholars. In Chapter 5, we explained our reasons behind conducting this work, and outlined how interviews were conducted and then analysed.

Then came the five StoryTeller chapters. In Chapter 6, Jo Mullen put forth an existential conceptualisation of creativity, arguing it is a natural "urge". Michelle McNary developed this in Chapter 7, with a reminder that sometimes the pressure of wanting to create but being unable to can add to distress. Chapter 8 was Peter Bullimore's view on just how important being creative has been for him on his own journey. Our anonymised actor ANON built on Michelle's ideas of creativity being a double-edged sword in Chapter 9, while also reminding us that creativity can have the power to "save". Anna Sexton was our final StoryTeller in Chapter 10, and gave a powerful account of how her creativity has gently allowed her to heal, and explored the idea of creative outputs as "artifacts" that are curated in our own personal narrative. Andrew Voyce then gave us an account of his own story in

DOI: 10.4324/9781003319405-13

Chapter 11, detailing how he moved from a diagnosis of schizophrenia to where he is today, and the role that creativity played in this.

In Chapter 12, Robert presented his analysis of the StoryTellers' interviews and outlined three key themes for creativity in recovery – as a psychological process, as a way of sense-making and socially. These were explored in detail, and from this a model was created to visualise the role of creativity in mental health recovery based upon the experiences of our StoryTellers. Finally, a table was created to suggest how on the back of this, creativity might need to be added to the CHIME framework as a distinct and significant factor in mental health recovery (Carson & Hurst, 2021). We hope that by presenting this analysis after the five StoryTeller chapters, we have humanised the frameworks and models drawn on and developed (Charlick et al., 2016).

This approach to exploring creativity was unique; prior Interpretative Phenomenological Analysis (IPA) studies of creativity and recovery have chosen to study it within the contexts of art-therapy (Deveney & Lawson, 2021), or daycentres (McDonnell, 2014). Rather than examining creativity within these contexts, this research stripped it back to the essential, individual experience – fully utilising the exploratory nature of IPA (Smith et al., 2009).

**Implications**

After the interviews, looking back on definitions of creativity which say that creative output must be "of value" (e.g., Andreasen, 2006) is concerning. Participants spoke about such social expectations being detrimental to their mental health. When creativity must have cultural worth, when there is a financial need to produce, the creativity can become toxic. Such definitions of creativity seem more in line with what was defined in Chapter 12 as "producing", or even "talent" or "success". Creativity, rather, is a free expression of the self. Creativity can be everyday, as is suggested elsewhere (Richards, 2010).

Acknowledging the potential inhibiting effects of social pressures fits with the philosophy of "Positive Psychology 2.0" (Wong, 2011). While creativity can be a force for good in recovery, this is not always the case. Exploring the negative aspects alongside the positives is important, to gain a holistic and realistic view.

This new suggested perspective on creativity in recovery is a first step. Further research is required before any level of policy change could be suggested. However, the model could be used to explain the process to those on recovery journeys, or to service providers.

The utopian outcome based on the findings of this research would be a societal change in the way that creativity is viewed. It requires emancipation, to the point where everyone can be aware of their instinctive and everyday creativity and then be able to utilise it. There was consensus among the StoryTellers that creativity is the origin of art, but not all creative artifacts need to be "art". Pressure around social judgement of creations was one of the key inhibitors of creativity. There is a need to separate the instinctive creative process from the end-product (Walia, 2019). How to achieve this is much more difficult. Further research, and then policy adjustments combined with public campaigns may help bring this ideal closer to reality.

While art therapies have been shown to be effective, it would be preferable for people to be encouraged to engage with their own instinctive creativity. Not every type of therapy will work for everyone. For example, while drama therapy can be beneficial for those with mental health diagnoses (Fernández-Aguayo & Pino-Juste, 2018), because of ANON's background in acting, and internalised standards of how it should be done, they may not reap the same reward as others. The present project demonstrated that being trained in a discipline tends to lead a person to internalise certain standards, and judge themselves harshly against these. In recommending art-based therapies, it is important to direct those in recovery towards therapies where there is an element of learning – this will minimise any frustrations at mistakes, and allow participants to be more in-tune with their instinctive creativity.

The need to understand personal limitations around creativity was a thread running through the interviews. This is important to understand for everybody. Peifer et al. (2020) found that having tasks unfinished at work had a negative impact on creativity levels for the rest of the day. Being able to formulate realistic expectations and manage self-expectations could lead to better wellbeing generally.

The study has shown that creativity is perhaps more significant to recovery than is currently acknowledged in academic spaces. While creative therapies can be useful, the sense from the interviews is that creativity is also a mindset, a philosophy for life. It can be a tool, too. Understanding the multi-faceted nature of creativity in further depth could help develop interventions to use in various contexts.

This could potentially be beneficial to those who are not in recovery. Non-clinical sample studies (e.g. Smernoff et al., 2019) often demonstrate that techniques or methods developed to help people recover often provide benefits to general populations too. The findings of this study, in regard to the *approach* shown to creativity by participants, could perhaps be beneficial in this way.

Finally, one of the outcomes of the study was a metaphor for "curating" creative outputs, or "artifacts". This metaphorical "museum" is a way of understanding the recovery journey so far through the things created at various points. This could perhaps be adapted into an intervention. There exist various guided interventions, whereby participants reflect on their values (Schippers & Ziegler, 2019) or write about their story so far (King et al., 2013). While these may be creative in that participants will craft a narrative, bringing previous creations, "artifacts", into consideration could be potentially highly beneficial.

### Suggestions for future research

Having further established the unique and personal nature of both creativity and recovery, it is difficult to recommend that future research tries to study how the two processes interact quantitatively. While doing so may provide a chance to understand the phenomenon with larger samples, the highly personal nature of both creativity and recovery would make this a difficult approach to take without losing richness and authenticity. While quantitative creativity measures exist and have been found to be able to predict wellbeing (Acar et al., 2021), these scales often focus on factors such as achievement (Carson et al., 2005). This is not in-line with the way that creativity seemed to be experienced in the recovery journey of our StoryTellers. They saw it as something not easily measured. Therefore, it is hard to understand what would be gained from such a study, outside of giving policy makers or service providers a set of numbers to instil them with confidence.

The previously discussed, potentially damaging definitions of creativity (e.g., Csikszentmihalyi, 1997) means that further work is required. The brief definition offered by this study could serve as a starting point for research which speaks to people with lived experience of creativity within recovery, to establish a more representative and psychological definition. If quantitative scales are to be used for assessing creativity, this project has highlighted a need to produce these based on lived experience of creativity, to prevent any confusion with concepts such as "talent" or "accomplishment".

All five participants had some issues with the language in and around recovery. Finding more appropriate terminology to use is important, to prevent those in recovery from feeling that their experiences are being colonised. This could be achieved through collaborative research between those with lived experience and researchers (Tomlinson & De Ruysscher, 2020).

Finally, with this project providing the proposed C-CHIME framework with some evidence, it requires further independent evidencing. This could be done through further qualitative analysis (Senneseth et al., 2022) or through application of the framework as an intervention assessed with quantitative measures (Ogilvie & Carson, 2023), with these methods utilised to look at adaptations of CHIME for forensic and addiction recovery purposes, respectively.

## Conclusions

### *Jerome*

It has been a pleasure to have worked on this book with Robert and Andrew. I have been fortunate to have worked on other projects with both men. One of the papers I am most proud of is the collaborative autoethnographic account I co-authored with Andrew about the time we were both at the University of Reading and our subsequent careers in psychiatry, but on opposite sides of the fence (Voyce & Carson, 2020). Andrew left Reading and entered a journey of becoming a "revolving door mental patient". In contrast, I embarked on a career in clinical psychology.

Andrew and I came together for the first-time years later through the writing of a book on psychosis (Cordle et al., 2011). Andrew later spoke at a conference held at the Institute of Psychiatry on his own journey and his remarkable recovery and also came to the book launch of the recovery heroes' book (Davies et al., 2011). After I left London, we lost touch. Yet every Christmas without fail, he would send me a Christmas card.

It was the COVID lockdown in 2020 that made me think maybe he could do a Zoom session for our students. Since then, he has presented on Zoom to a variety of students. Patrick Hopkinson and I then hit on the idea of comparing Andrew's mental health recovery with that of the musician Syd Barrett of Pink Floyd (Hopkinson et al., 2021). We were later joined by Mats Niklasson and Peter Bryngelsson, and co-authored further papers on Peter Green (Fleetwood Mac) and Brian Wilson (the Beach Boys) (Hopkinson et al., 2022, 2023). Andrew and I are hoping to give a joint presentation to psychology students at Reading in late 2024, which will be a career highlight for both of us. A kind of "going home".

Robert did his undergraduate project under my supervision. He looked at the topic of meaning in life (Hurst & Carson, 2021c). We are both proud of our first collaborative autoethnographic paper (Hurst & Carson, 2021a). Robert then started studying the Remarkable Lives set of papers, which led him to deduce that while there was evidence for the CHIME framework, all of the contributors were also highly creative individuals and hence there was a need to expand the framework to C-CHIME (Carson & Hurst, 2021; Hurst & Carson, 2021b; Hurst et al., 2022). Robert went onto to explore the link between creativity and recovery for his MSc dissertation, which I again supervised. It was only natural that Robert would take over the Remarkable Lives series (detailed in Chapter 3), which he has successfully done.

This book presents the narratives of five amazing individuals, all of whom have been able to use creativity in their own unique ways to lead more fulfilling lives, despite enduring mental health problems. Their accounts are inspiring. I am sure each of them will continue to achieve great things in their lives and make a difference. I have collated living tributes for Andrew (Carson, 2024a) and for Peter Bullimore (Carson, 2024b) to show the impact that both men have made in the field of mental health with many people. It is my hope that Andrew, Robert, and I will be able to continue our academic work for many years to come and that we continue to develop autoethnographic approaches to helping people learn more about mental health and what truly helps people flourish (Seligman, 2011) and not languish (Keyes, 2024), such as creativity. That is my dream.

### Andrew

I want to be treated like a human being.

(Spiegelman, 1988, p. 56)

The five StoryTellers want the same. Their stories are their own: the five interviewees all presented an individual and provocative storyline. This collective debate around the validity of definitions of recovery and creativity, and how they should be applied, is a hallmark of the unexpected arising from qualitative methodology.

Two themes that emerge from the discussion of recovery in Chapter 12 are that there is personal determination and meaning around a journey where you do not necessarily get back to somewhere you were before; and that there is scepticism around the institutionalisation of recovery, especially in clinical practice. As

Repper and Perkins (2003, p. 13) remark: "[There are raised] important questions about the relative status of different sorts of expertise – the expertise of personal experience versus the expertise of degrees and qualifications".

The value judgements of others mitigate against the individual's ownership of their narrative, as is mentioned in Chapter 11. From an individual questioning of the concept and location of recovery practice, is joined a meta-discussion of an ethical and power-relations perspective. Who owns the practice of mental health recovery?

This book gives a platform to the voices of all five interviewees and three co-authors. In particular, these combined voices mitigate against being othered, marginalised, or excluded. There is indeed a broad range of discussion in this book around creativity and recovery. Michelle and ANON caution against burnout during the creative process, but it is clear from the combined voices of the StoryTellers that they have taken control of their narratives. A question might be to enquire if others, in particular mental health professionals, have put forward a version of who the interviewees are. From the re-authoring of their stories will emerge their own identity that they are happy to live with. Recognition of a person's creative output is essential as creativity is intertwined with the self, and is constructed by that self, not someone else. This is a theme for all five StoryTellers.

It is a hugely useful exercise to revisit these points on a journey, especially if one has suffered through mental difficulties or through contact with the mental health system. "There is no greater agony than bearing an untold story inside", Maya Angelou is said to have written, and to re-author one's narrative as the five StoryTellers have done is essential to wellbeing. A gateway to a sense of identity. Their stories are included in their respective chapters, but also in their creative activities. They need not explicitly be stories about mental health.

There is a value in reflection and the unexpected opinions around recovery and creativity in this book, making one challenge views that seem innate in the understanding of the aftermath of poor mental health. It may not be as one assumes, there can be a process of learning from the five StoryTellers. It is healthy to question beliefs and to avoid acceptance of what is there, merely because it is there. The StoryTellers between them have challenged the notion of recovery and have a diverse understanding of creativity. There is a liberation arising from disputing what makes recovery, whether recovery is the right interpretation of where StoryTellers are going; and if creativity has to fit into narrow definitions.

"You just need to figure out your own path with it" (ANON); "I … accepted subconsciously that it was something that I would have to work through" (Anna). In their way, the StoryTellers are using their creativity to challenge and to liberate themselves from stereotypes.

Where does this put definitions of recovery and the healing attributes of creative endeavour? Does the personal resistance to being pigeon-holed have a more widespread resonance? These questions can be resolved by listening to the individual's voice and accepting little narratives while rejecting grand narratives (Sim & Van Loon, 2009). Recovery is a rebellion against the medical model and yet also contains the seeds of a rejection of itself too, as expressed by the StoryTellers.

Regarding the power relations involved with this, Michel Foucault identified a binary of power and marginalisation, where the marginalisation of those with mental health challenges enables the operation of power (Sim & Van Loon, 2009, p. 94). In eschewing their voices, the operation of power by others in their lives can have the effect of usurping their stories from those with mental health challenges.

Having a voice provides a model of resistance and liberation.

So, where the very notion of recovery is put up for discussion by the five StoryTellers, by giving their version of their own narrative, the least that can be said is that their voices are heard. None of the five subscribe to a meta-theory, but they are clear on their own personal narratives and how creativity has enabled their journeys. Creative journeys of discovery that are intertwined with ownership, independence, and autonomy.

### *Robert*

We started this book with several examples of creativity – many of these were examples from people in captivity. This was useful to us narratively, as being physically imprisoned is a physical manifestation of how it can be to be separated from society, as those with lived experience often can be due to stigma. Extreme and concrete examples of adversity. They also showed the possible emancipatory nature of creativity. It is one of the last personal things that can be taken from us. We can all hum a tune in our head, even in dire circumstances. In these examples, the creativity was innate, instinctive. It wasn't suggested by medical professionals.

Is the current culture of creativity in itself imprisoning? There is this sense that any creativity must become a commodity. Everyday (little-c) creativity is therefore rebellion. Doing it for fun or expression is breaking the trend. Creativity needs to be emancipated from limiting definitions, from expectations of how it should look, from lack of access to resources.

In Chapter 5, I mentioned witnessing some inspiring examples of creativity-as-rebellion while in Estonia. After a short ferry across the Baltic Sea to Helsinki, Finland, I was awestruck by the recently constructed public library there. As well as a bright and inviting marvel of architecture made *for people*, the contents within blew me away. With free-to-use sewing machines, 3D printers, even recording studios, to my mind it serves as a blueprint for how creativity can be further democratised. While people still need to be given time to pursue creative interests, providing the physical resources publicly is an incredible step towards making creativity more accessible.

In Estonia, I saw a glimpse from the past of how supressing and suffocating people does not prevent their creativity from causing cracks, from breaking through. In Helsinki, the opposite was acting out in real time as people sat at equipment and created – an open and nurturing meadow of possibility provided to the people.

A question that I have grappled with throughout this project is "are current definitions of creativity (both in psychological literature and the public discourse) helpful?". I have tried to understand creativity beyond ideas of talent and success, strip it back to its essential nature to understand what role it can play for people in their darkest days. We have seen that this version of creativity can be a saving grace.

In Chapter 5, I alluded to John Berger's *Ways of Seeing* being a major inspiration for me. In the book adapted from the series, Berger's foreword ends with the line "Our principal aim has been to start a process of questioning" (Berger, 2008, p. 5). I hope to have achieved a similar aim with this work. To have inspired readers to question the way they view creativity – their own, and that of others.

For the five StoryTellers who make up the backbone of this project, creativity was a big part of not just their recovery journeys but their lives as a whole. It was an escape, a tool for recovery, a philosophy. It is essential. It "saves".

## References

Acar, S., Tadik, H., Myers, D., Van der Sman, C., & Uysal, R. (2021). Creativity and well-being: A meta-analysis. *The Journal of Creative Behavior*, *55*(*3*), 738–751. doi:10.1002/jocb.485.

Andreasen, N. C. (2006). *The creative brain: The science of genius*. Plume.

Berger, J. (2008). *Ways of seeing*. Penguin.

Carson, J. (2024a). Andrew Voyce: A living tribute. "You can end up in a happy place." *Mental Health and Social Inclusion*, *28*(*3*), 208–222. doi:10.1108/MHSI-04-2023-0046.

Carson, J. (2024b). Peter Bullimore: A living tribute. *Mental Health and Social Inclusion*, *28*(*1*), 17–29. doi:10.1108/MHSI-04-2023-0038.

Carson, J., & Hurst, R. (2021). Mental health nursing and recovery: The C-CHIME model. *British Journal of Mental Health Nursing*, *10*(*2*), 1–3. doi:10.12968.bjmh.2021.0011.

Carson, S. H., Peterson, J. B., & Higgins, D. M. (2005). Reliability, validity, and factor structure of the creative achievement questionnaire. *Creativity Research Journal*, *17*(*1*), 37–50. doi:10.1207/s15326934crj1701_4.

Charlick, S., Pincombe, J., McKellar, L., & Fielder, A. (2016). Making sense of participant experiences: Interpretative phenomenological analysis in midwifery research. *International Journal of Doctoral Studies*, *11*, 205–216. https://www.informingscience.org/Publications/3486.

Cordle, H., Fradgley, J., Carson, J., Holloway, F., & Richards, P. (Eds.). (2011). *Psychosis: Stories of recovery and hope*. Quay Publishers.

Csikszentmihalyi, M. (1997). *Creativity: The psychology of discovery and invention*. HarperCollins.

Davies, S., Wakely, E., Morgan, S., & Carson, J. (Eds.) (2011). *Mental health recovery heroes past and present: A handbook for mental healthcare staff, service users and carers*. Pavilion.

Deveney, C., & Lawson, P. (2021). Writing your way to well-being: An IPA analysis of the therapeutic effects of creative writing on mental health and the processing of emotional difficulties. *Counselling and Psychotherapy Research*, *22*(*2*), 292–300. doi:10.1002/capr.12435.

Fernández-Aguayo, S., & Pino-Juste, M. (2018). Drama therapy and theater as an intervention tool: Bibliometric analysis of programs based on drama therapy and theater. *The Arts in Psychotherapy*, *59*, 83–93. doi:10.1016/j.aip.2018.04.001.

Hopkinson, P., Bryngelsson, P., Voyce, A., Niklasson, M., & Carson, J. (2022). A tale of two Peters: An analysis of the life of Peter Green using collaborative/community autoethnography and digital team ethnography. *Mental Health and Social Inclusion*, *27(1)*, 3–19. doi:10.1108/MHSI-09-2022-0062.

Hopkinson, P., Niklasson, M., Bryngelsson, P., Voyce, A., & Carson, J. (2023). Not so good vibrations: Five collaborative autoethnographic accounts of Brian Wilson, his life, music, rock 'n' recovery. *Mental Health and Social Inclusion*, *27(4)*, 430–446. doi:10.1108/MHSI-09-2023-0103.

Hopkinson, P., Voyce, A., & Carson, J. (2021). Syd Barrett took a left turn and never came back. Andrew Voyce did. Why? *Mental Health and Social Inclusion*, *25(4)*. 385–395. doi:10-1108/MHSI-06-2021-00031.

Hurst, R., & Carson, J. (2021a). Be honest: Why did YOU decide to study psychology? A recent graduate and a professor reflect. *Psychology Teaching Review*, *27(2)*, 22–35.

Hurst, R., & Carson, J. (2021b). For whom the bell chimes: A synthesis of remarkable student lives. *Mental Health and Social Inclusion*, *25(2)*, 195–207. doi:10.1108/MHSI-10-2020-0071.

Hurst, R., & Carson, J. (2021c). Stressing the meaning: A quantitative study of the effects of meaning in life and depression on academic stress in psychology undergraduates. *International Journal of Existential Positive Psychology*, *10(1)*, 1–14.

Hurst, R., Carson, J., Shahama, A., Kay, H., Nabb, C., & Prescott, J. (2022) Remarkable recoveries: An interpretation of recovery narratives using the CHIME Model. *Mental Health and Social Inclusion*, *26(2)*, 175–190. doi:10.1108/MHSI-01-2022-0001.

Keyes, C. (2024). *Languishing: How to feel alive again in a world that wears us down.* Penguin Random House.

King, R., Neilsen, P., & White, E. (2013). Creative writing in recovery from severe mental illness. *International Journal of Mental Health Nursing*, *22(5)*, 444–452. doi:10.1111/j.1447-0349.2012.00891.x.

Leamy, M., Bird, V., Le Boutillier, C., Williams, J., & Slade, M. (2011). Conceptual framework for personal recovery in mental health: Systematic review and narrative synthesis. *The British Journal of Psychiatry*, *199(6)*, 445–452. doi:10.1192/bjp.bp.110.083733.

McDonnell, R. (2014). *Creativity and social support in mental health: Service users' perspectives.* Springer.

Ogilvie, L., & Carson, J. (2023). Positive addiction recovery therapy: A replication and follow-up study. *Advances in Dual Diagnosis*, *16(4)*, 227–241. doi:10.1108/ADD-05-2023-0010.

Peifer, C., Syrek, C., Ostwald, V., Schuh, E., & Antoni, C. H. (2020). Thieves of flow: How unfinished tasks at work are related to flow experience and wellbeing. *Journal of Happiness Studies*, *21(5)*, 1641–1660. doi:10.1007/s10902-019-00149-z.

Repper, J., & Perkins, R. (2003). *Social inclusion and recovery.* Balliere Tindall.

Richards, R. (2010). Everyday creativity: Process and way of life – four key issues. In J. C. Kaufman & R. J. Sternberg (Eds.), *The Cambridge handbook of creativity* (pp. 189–215). Cambridge University Press. doi:10.1017/CBO9780511763205.013.

Schippers, M. C., & Ziegler, N. (2019). Life crafting as a way to find purpose and meaning in life. *Frontiers in Psychology*, *10*. doi:10.3389/fpsyg.2019.02778.

Seligman, M. (2011). *Flourish.* Nicholas Brealey.

Senneseth, M., Pollak, C., Urheim, R., Logan, C., & Palmstierna, T. (2022). Personal recovery and its challenges in forensic mental health: Systematic review and thematic synthesis of the qualitative literature. *BJPsych Open*, *8(1)*, e17. doi:10.1192/bjo.2021.1068.

Sim, S., & Van Loon, B. (2009). *Introducing critical theory: A graphic guide.* Icon Books.

Smernoff, E., Mitnik, I., & Lev-Ari, S. (2019). The effects of inquiry-based stress reduction (IBSR) on mental health and well-being among a non-clinical sample. *Complementary Therapies in Clinical Practice*, *34*, 30–34. doi:10.1016/j.ctcp.2018.10.015.

Smith, J. A., Flowers, P., & Larkin, M. (2009). *Interpretative phenomenological analysis: Theory, method and research.* Sage Publications.

Spiegelman, A. (1988). *Maus.* Penguin.

Tomlinson, P., & De Ruysscher, C. (2020). From monologue to dialogue in mental health care research: Reflections on a collaborative research process. *Disability & Society, 35(8)*, 1274–1289. doi:10.1080/09687599.2019.1680345.

Voyce, A., & Carson, J. (2020). Our lives in three parts: An autoethnographic account of two undergraduates and their respective psychiatric careers. *Mental Health and Social Inclusion, 24(4)*, 197–205. doi:10.1108/MHSI-07-2020-0045.

Walia, C. (2019). A dynamic definition of creativity. *Creativity Research Journal, 31(3)*, 237–247. doi:10.1080/10400419.2019.1641787.

Wong, P. T. (2011). Positive psychology 2.0: Towards a balanced interactive model of the good life. *Canadian Psychology/Psychologie Canadienne, 52(2)*, 69–81. doi:10.1037/a0022511.

# Index

For Product Safety Concerns and Information please contact our EU
representative  GPSR@taylorandfrancis.com
Taylor & Francis Verlag GmbH, Kaufingerstraße 24, 80331 München, Germany

www.ingramcontent.com/pod-product-compliance
Lightning Source LLC
Chambersburg PA
CBHW052010270326
41929CB00015B/2857

9 7 8 1 0 3 2 3 3 3 6 8 7